All About Insulin

More Than 400 Frequently Asked Questions From Real Patients

By

Shunzhong Shawn Bao, MD

Medical Editor: Richard Rapp, MD

Editor: Barbara Winter

Ace Health Publisher

Publisher's Note/Disclaimer

The information contained herein is not intended to replace the services of a trained health professional or to be a substitute for individual medical advice. You should consult with your healthcare professional regarding to any matter related to your health, and in particular, any matter that may require diagnosis and medical attention.

The misuse of insulin can be very dangerous and sometimes can be life-threatening, which can hurt you and other people. For your specific condition or situation and individualized treatment target, plan, specific procedure and protocols, you need to consult your healthcare team. Therefore, the author, editor, or publisher cannot assume any responsibility for harm caused by any information presented in this book.

First Edition 2018

All About Insulin

More Than 400 Frequently Asked Questions From Real Patients

Shunzhong Shawn Bao, MD

Richard Rapp, Medical Editor

Barbara Winter, Editor

Published by Ace Health Publisher

Dedication

This book is dedicated to my patients. These are their intelligent questions for which I am grateful. They motivate me to think, continue learning and improving my patient care every day. These days, doctors do not have enough time to address all the questions patients may have, so I hope my patients can get the answers they need from this book.

I want to thank my nurses, Betty Westbury and Carla Stacks who are providing excellent care to my patients and are first readers of this book. With their critiques, they have made significant contributions to this book.

In addition, this book is also dedicated to my good friend, my editor, Barbara Winter, and her unending kindness and generosity. With her patience and critical editing, she has made this book readable.

This book is dedicated to my best friend, my medical editor, Dr. Richard Rapp. He has spent countless hours reviewing every question in this book. We have discussed different options and answers, and some of them have been completely rewritten for accuracy and clarity. He has made significant contributions to this book.

Finally, this book is dedicated to my wife who deserves deep, enduring gratitude, and to my two children who are both in medical school, studying and working very hard. They inspire me to learn and strive for excellence in patient care.

Preface

"Insulin is one of the greatest scientific discoveries, but using it is not a science; it is an art." –My patient

Insulin has become the mainstream treatment for both type I and type II diabetes, as well other diabetes. Many patients have been started on insulin but have not received adequate education about the art involved in its use. I have seen patients misuse insulin, causing severe fluctuations of sugar and significant weight gain; I have seen patients mistitrate insulin and use one thousand units of insulin a day; I have seen patients end up in a "vegetative state" due to insulin misuse. Many patients are using one of the most dangerous medications without proper education.

Diabetes is complicated. My experience has shown that patients who make sustainable lifestyle changes will do the best. I published a book <<Diabetes Questions and Answers, More Than 400 Frequently Asked Questions>> (available on Amazon.com and in all major bookstores), where I answer real questions from my patients. I emphasize the non-starch plant-based diet and daily exercise. Some of my patients have been able to lose half of their body weight using my diet and exercise recommendations. We have been able to reverse prediabetes and put diabetes into remission. Insulin should not be the only answer. I recommend the diet and exercise lifestyle to optimize diabetes control, before ramping insulin dosage to get control. I have patients coming to me on a high dose of insulin and reasonable HbA1C. The doctor might get the patient to believe that the diabetes is under control because A1c is good. The reality is that the patient has frequent hypoglycemia, which might cause a heart attack, stroke and increase mortality. It is true. Sugar is fluctuating, but we want it to be as little as possible.

This book <<All about insulin>> answers more than 400 questions from real patients about insulin. These are your questions and my answers. There are many ways to deal with one situation. In the book, I provide my way in dealing with the problem. Your doctor might provide different solution. Before you apply my recommendation, you always need to discuss it with your physician.

Again, insulin is very complicated and dangerous. I hope you can use it artfully for your benefit. Keep learning. Knowledge is power. If you are determined, you will be better.

If you have a question about insulin which is not in this book, please write to me. I might be able to include it in the next edition.

Table of Contents

CHAPTER 1. GENERAL INFORMATION ABOUT STARTING INSULIN 3

What basic information should I know before starting insulin injections? 3

Where can I inject? 5

Which one is better? Pen or vial? 6

Which needle is better? 6

What are the potential short-term adverse effects? 6

What are the potential long-term adverse effects of insulin? 7

What can I expect after I start insulin injection? 7

What if some insulin leaks back out of the injection site? 9

What should I do if there is bleeding or bruising at the injection site? 10

What should I do if I have injection site redness and itchiness? 10

What happens if you accidentally inject too much insulin? 10

What happens if an air bubble was accidentally injected? 11

Can I reuse my needles or syringes? 11

Can I leave the needle on the pen (after I have already used this needle for a prior injection) to be used for new injection? 11

I have type 2 diabetes, and I was recommended to start insulin. Does it mean I have to be on insulin forever? 11

I have type 2 diabetes, why should I start insulin? 12

What precautions must I take if I am using insulin and driving? 12

Which type of insulin is best? 13

What is long-acting insulin(basal insulin)? 13

What is short-acting insulin (rapid-acting insulin, fast-acting insulin)? 13

Are there any other types of insulin? 14

Who can use inhaled insulin? 19

What should I do if I forget to take my long-acting insulin (basal insulin, slow-acting insulin)? 19

What should I do if I accidentally inject short-acting insulin for long-acting insulin? 22

What should I do if I accidentally inject long-acting insulin (slow-acting, basal insulin) for short-acting insulin (fast-acting, rapid-acting insulin)? 23

What should I do if I accidentally inject myself with long-acting as short-acting and short-acting as long-acting? 27

I was prescribed basal insulin two times a day, and the morning dose is so much more than night dose. I injected the morning dose at night. What should I do? 28

Why is pre-mixed insulin not optimal for type 1 diabetes? 29

Why are some insulins clear and other insulins cloudy? 30

How should I store insulin? 30

I do not have a good memory. I think I gave myself a shot a minute ago, but I am not sure if I did or did not. Is there anything I can do? 31

What else do I need to remember when I do an injection? 32

If I have type 2 diabetes, what can I do to prevent weight gain with insulin use? 32

Can you tell me more about basal and bolus regimen? 34

Do you have general tips on how to use fixed or scheduled dose insulin regimen? 35

What is a sliding scale? How do I use it? 38

Can you give me some examples of the sliding scale (correction scale)? 38

I have type 1 diabetes. Do you have general recommendations about how to adjust long-acting insulin? 44

I have type 2 diabetes. Do you have a general recommendation about how to adjust long-acting insulin? 45

My previous doctor recommended I not change my basal insulin dose. What is your rationale behind adjusting my basal insulin dose? 46

Is there an app to help me calculate my insulin dosage? 47

What should I do with those needles and sharps? 47

What is a proposed target of sugar and A1c? 47

Can I have a personalized day to day dose adjustment guideline? 51

CHAPTER 2. GLARGINE: LANTUS/BASAGLAR **55**

What is Lantus? What is Basaglar?.. 55

I have type 2 diabetes. My doctor started me on Lantus (or biosimilar Basaglar). Should I give it in the morning or night, before a meal or after a meal? 55

I have type 2 diabetes. My doctor wanted to start me on Lantus (or biosimilar Basaglar). What is the appropriate starting dose?............. 56

I have type 2 diabetes, my doctor wanted to start me on Lantus (or biosimilar Basaglar), what is your recommendation for titrating the dose? 56

I have type 2 diabetes, and my doctor started me on Lantus or Basaglar once a day. How often should I check my sugar?................................. 57

Do you recommend vial or pen?.. 57

If I am using the pen, can I leave the needle on for the next injection? 57

If I use the pen, should I leave the pen in the refrigerator or room temperature? 57

After I start to use the pen, how long can I use it?.............................. 58

If I use the vial, can I put the vial back in the refrigerator after using it? 58

If I start to use the vial, how long can I use it? 58

How long can I store unopened pens and vials?................................... 58

How can I transport insulin?... 58

I am using Lantus or Basaglar, but my morning sugar is still way too high. What can I do? 58

I am on Lantus/Basaglar, and my morning sugar is too low. What should I do? 59

I want to eat a big meal, can I give more Lantus or Basaglar? 60

I was hospitalized recently; the hospital used Levemir on me, but I have Lantus (or Basaglar) at home. What should I do?............................... 60

My insurance changed my coverage from Levemir to Lantus or Basaglar. What can I do? 61

I was using Humulin N (Novolin N) two times a day. Now my doctor has changed it to Lantus or Basaglar. What should I do?.......................... 61

I am on premixed insulin (like Novolin 70/30, Humulin 70/30, Humalog 75/25, Humalog 50/50, Novolog 70/30), and now my doctor wants to switch me to Lantus or Basaglar. What should I do? 62

My insurance wants me to change Lantus to Basaglar. What should I do?... 62

My insurance wants me to change Toujeo to Lantus or Basaglar. What can I do? 62

My insurance wants me to change from Tresiba to Lantus or Basaglar. What should I do? 63

What else is in Lantus?.. 63

What is m-cresol? Is it toxic?... 63

What is polysorbate-20? Is it toxic? 64

Should I stop Lantus since it contains toxic substances?...... 64

If I am allergic to Lantus or Basaglar, what options do I have? 64

CHAPTER 3. GLARGINE: TOUJEO **67**

What is Toujeo?... 67

Is Toujeo better than Lantus or Basaglar?............................. 67

I have type 2 diabetes and my doctor started me on Toujeo. Should I give it in the morning or night? 67

I have type 2 diabetes, and my doctor wanted to start me on Toujeo. What is the appropriate starting dose? 68

I have type 2 diabetes and my doctor wanted to start me on Toujeo, what is your recommendation for titrating the dose? 69

I was started on Toujeo, and now I am pregnant. What should I do?.. 69

Do you recommend vial or pen?... 70

If I am using the pen, can I leave the needle on for the next injection? 70

Should I leave the Toujeo pen in the refrigerator or outside at room temperature? 70

After I start a new pen, how long can I use it?...................... 70

How long can I store the unopened pens of Toujeo?............. 70

How can I transport insulin Toujeo?...................................... 71

I am using Toujeo but my morning sugar is still way too high. What can I do?.. 71

I want to eat a big meal. Can I give more Toujeo? 71

I was hospitalized recently and the hospital used Lantus/or Basaglar or Levemir on me, but I use Toujeo at home. What should I do?.............. 72

My insurance changed my coverage from Lantus, Basaglar, or Levemir to Toujeo. What can I do? 72

I was using Humulin N (Novolin N) 2 times a day. Now my doctor changed it to Toujeo. What should I do?.................... 72

I am on a premix insulin like Novolin 70/30, Humulin 70/30, Humalog 75/25, Novolog 70/30, and now my doctor wants to switch me to Toujeo. What should I do?.................... 73

My insurance wants me to change from Tresiba to Toujeo. What should I do?.................... 74

What else is in Toujeo?.................... 74

What is m-cresol? Is it toxic?.................... 74

Should I stop Toujeo since it contains toxic substances?.................... 75

If I am allergic to Toujeo, what options do I have?.................... 75

CHAPTER 4 : LEVEMIR.................... **77**

What is Levemir?.................... 77

I have type 2 diabetes and my doctor started me on Levemir. Should I give it in the morning or night?.................... 77

I have type 2 diabetes and my doctor wanted to start me on Levemir. What is the appropriate starting dose?.................... 78

I have type 2 diabetes and my doctor wants to start me on Levemir. What is your recommendation for titrating the dose?.................... 78

Do you recommend vial or pen?.................... 78

After I start using a new pen, how long can I use it?.................... 79

If I use the vial, can I put the vial back in the refrigerator after each use?.................... 79

If I start to use the vial, how long can I use it?.................... 79

How long can I store the unopened pens and vials?.................... 79

How can I transport Levemir?.................... 79

I am using Levemir and my morning sugar is still way too high. What should I do?.................... 79

I want to eat a big meal, can I give more Levemir?.................... 80

I was hospitalized recently and the hospital used Lantus or Basaglar on me, but I use Levemir at home. What should I do?.................... 80

My insurance changed my coverage from Lantus or Basaglar to Levemir. What can I do?.................... 81

I was using Humulin N (Novolin N) twice a day. Now my doctor has changed it to Levemir. What should I do?.................... 81

I am on premix insulin like Novolin 70/30, Humulin 70/30, Humalog 75/25, Humalog 50/50, or Novolog 70/30, and now my doctor wants to switch me to Levemir. What should I do?.. 81

My insurance wants me to change from Toujeo to Levemir. What can I do?.. 82

My insurance wants me to change from Tresiba to Levemir. What should I do? 83

What else is in Levemir?... 83

What is m-cresol? Is it toxic?.. 83

What is mannitol? Is it toxic? 84

Should I stop Levemir since it contains toxic substance?.................... 84

If I am allergic to Levemir, what options do I have?............................. 84

CHAPTER 5 : TRESIBA...**85**

What is Tresiba?... 85

Should I give it in the morning or night? 85

I have type 2 diabetes, and my doctor wants to start me on Tresiba. What is the appropriate starting dose? 85

I have type 2 diabetes and my doctor wanted to start me on Tresiba. What is your recommendation for titrating the dose?......................... 86

Do you recommend a vial or pen?... 86

For some reason, I have both U-100 and U-200 pens. What should I pay attention to when I do the injection? 87

If I am using the pen, can I leave the needle on for the next injection? 87

If I use the pen, should I leave the pen in the refrigerator or at room temperature? 87

After I start using a new pen, how long can I use it?............................ 87

How long can I store the unopened pens? 87

How long can I store the unopened pen at room temperature?.......... 88

How can I transport Tresiba insulin?.. 88

I am using Tresiba and my morning sugar is still way too high............ 88

I want to eat a big meal. Can I give more Tresiba? 89

I was hospitalized recently, and the hospital used Lantus, Basaglar or Levemir on me. I have Tresiba at home. What should I do?............... 89

My insurance changed my coverage from Lantus, Basaglar, or Levemir to Tresiba. What can I do? 89

I was using Humulin N (Novolin N) twice a day and now my doctor has changed it to Tresiba. What should I do? 90

I am on premix insulin like Novolin 70/30, Humulin 70/30, Humalog 75/25, or Novolog 70/30, and now my doctor wants to switch me to Tresiba. What should I do? 90

My insurance wants me to change from Toujeo to Tresiba. What can I do? 91

My insurance wants me to change from Levemir to Tresiba. What should I do? 91

What else is in Tresiba? 92

What is metacresol (m-cresol)? Is it toxic? 92

Should I stop Tresiba since it contains toxic substances? 93

If I am allergic to Tresiba, what options do I have? 93

CHAPTER 6. NPH (HUMULIN N OR NOVOLIN N) **95**

What is NPH (Humulin N or Novolin N)? 95

I have type 2 diabetes and my doctor started me on NPH (N). Should I give it in the morning or night? 95

I have type 2 diabetes and my doctor wants to start me on NPH (N). What is the appropriate starting dose? 96

I have type 2 diabetes and my doctor wanted to start me on NPH (N). What is your recommendation for titrating the dose? 96

Do you recommend vial or pen? 97

If I am using the pen, can I leave the needle on for the next injection? 97

If I use the pen, should I leave the pen in the refrigerator or at room temperature? 97

How long can I store the unopened pens and vials? 98

How long can I store the unopened vial or pen at room temperature? 98

How long can I store a vial or pen in use? 98

How can I transport NPH insulin? 99

I am using NPH and my morning sugar is still way too high. What should I do? 99

I am using NPH and my morning sugar is too low. What should I do? 100

I want to eat a big meal, so can I give more NPH? 101

I was hospitalized recently and the hospital used Lantus or Basaglar (or Levemir) on me, but I have NPH at home and am not able to afford any other insulin. What should I do?.. 101

My insurance changed my coverage. Now it doesn't pay for any Lantus or Basaglar, Tresiba, Toujeo or Levemir. What can I do?.................... 102

Can I mix my NPH with regular insulin? 102

How do I mix my NPH and regular insulin or other short-acting insulin? 102

Can I mix any other insulin with NPH?... 105

What else is in NPH?.. 105

What is metacresol (m-cresol)? Is it toxic?.. 106

Should I stop NPH since it contains toxic substances?....................... 106

If I am allergic to NPH, what options do I have? 106

I am traveling and I ran out of my prescription. What can I do?........ 107

I have type 1 diabetes, and I have severe fluctuating sugar. What should I do? 107

I have type 2 diabetes. Can you give me some guidelines on adjusting my dose of NPH? 107

What you proposed above is too complicated. I tried it, my sugar is still up and down. What can I do?... 109

CHAPTER 7. HUMULIN R U-500 111

What is U-500 insulin?... 111

When do we use U-500?... 111

Who are the typical patients currently treated with U-500?............. 111

Why do you avoid prescribing U-500?... 111

Do I need to do some conversion with U-500 insulin pen?................. 113

I was prescribed U-500 vial and tuberculin syringes. However, I could not get tuberculin syringes. What can I do?... 113

Can I use U-500 in an insulin pump? 114

Can I mix U-500 and U-100 insulin and do one injection?................. 114

How long can I store U-500 insulin?.. 114

What else is in U-500 human insulin? 114

What is m-cresol? Is it toxic?.. 115

Should I stop U-500 since it contains toxic substance? 115

How can I titrate my U-500 insulin dose?.. 115

CHAPTER 8. INHALED INSULIN **117**

What is inhaled insulin? 117

Who can use it? 117

Who cannot use it? 117

What is the advantage of using Afrezza? 118

How should Afrezza be stored? 118

What is the dosage form? 118

What is the common adverse reaction? 118

What are the warnings and precautions? 118

I have never been on premeal insulin. At what dose should I start? .. 119

I have been taking premeal insulin. How do I convert? 119

How do I titrate on Afrezza dose? 119

What is the maximum dose? 120

Do I need a pen to be prepared just in case? 120

When should I temporarily hold my Afrezza? 120

CHAPTER 9. LONG-ACTING INSULIN AND GLP-1 AGONIST COMBINATION
.... **121**

What is Soliqua 100/33? 121

What is glargine? 121

What is GLP-1 agonist? 121

What does the 100/33 following Soliqua mean? 122

Is lixisenatide also available by itself? 122

What is Xultophy 100/3.6? 122

What does the number 100/3.6 mean after Xultophy? 122

What is the benefit of using GLP-1 agonist in diabetics? 122

*Why do we use a combination of long-acting insulin and a GLP-1
agonist?* 123

What is the disadvantage of taking the combination? 123

What else in Soliqua 100/33 besides glargine and lixisenatide? 124

*Who should not take the combination long-acting insulin and GLP-1
agonists?* 124

*When should I temporarily hold or permanently stop Soliqua 100/33 or
Xultophy 100/3.6?* 125

What are other possible adverse side effects? 126

When should I take it? 126

What can I do if I miss my dose? 126

How should I store Soliqua 100/33 or Xultophy 100/3.6? 127

How can I adjust my doses of Soliqua 100/33? 128

How can I adjust my dose of Xultophy 100/3.6? 129

What should I do if I use the maximum dose, but my sugar is still high?

.... 130

CHAPTER 10. FAST-ACTING INSULIN ANALOGS **131**

What is Humalog? 131

What are the dose forms for Humalog? 131

How fast? How long does it work after being subcutaneously injected?

.... 132

What else is in Humalog? 132

What is the difference between Humalog U-100 and U-200? 132

Who should consider the Humalog U-200 pen? 133

I was switched from Humalog U-100 to U-200. Do I need any conversion

factor? 133

Why do I need Humalog U-200? 133

What should I do if I overdose myself with fast-acting insulin? 134

My insurance wants me to change from Apidra, Novolog to Humalog.

What can I do? 135

My insurance does not pay for analog (Apidra, Novolog, Humalog)

anymore. What can I do? 135

What is Novolog? 135

What are the dosage forms? 136

What is the difference between Novolog and Humalog? 136

My insurance switched me from Humalog to Novolog. What should I

do? 136

What are the storage instructions for Novolog? 137

What are the ingredients in Novolog? 137

What is Apidra? 137

What are the dose forms for Apidra? 138

How fast and how long does Apidra work after being subcutaneously

injected? 138

What else is in Apidra? 138

My insurance wants me to change from Humalog or Novolog to Apidra. What can I do? 138

What is Fiasp? 138

What is the clinical advantage of Fiasp? 139

What else in Fiasp? 139

How fast and how long does Fiasp work after being subcutaneously injected? 139

How is Fiasp supplied? 140

How is Fiasp stored? 140

I am pregnant. Can I continue to use Fiasp? 140

My doctor change me to Humalog, Novolog, Apidra to Fiasp. What should I do? 140

I am allergic to Fiasp. What can I do? 141

CHAPTER 11. REGULAR INSULIN (NOVOLIN R AND HUMULIN R) 143

What is the difference between insulin R and analogs (Humalog, Novolog, Apidra, Fiasp)? 143

Why do we use analogs more than regular R? 143

Are there any situation where insulin R is preferred? 143

Where can I get the lowest price? 144

Can I get insulin R in a pen? 144

My insurance does not pay for analogs (Humalog, Novolog, or Apidra). What can I do? 144

Can I mix insulin R with other insulin? 145

CHAPTER 12. PREMIX INSULIN 147

What are the premix insulins? 147

What are the regular premix insulins on the market? 147

Are there any differences between the Humulin premix and Novolin premix? 148

What should I know if I am going to use Humulin premix and Novolin premix? 148

How should I store my regular premix insulin vial? 148

How should I store my regular premix insulin pen? 149

What are the newer versions of premix insulin (analog premix insulin)? 149

Is the newer version mix better than the regular premix insulin? 149

How should the newer premix insulin vial be stored? 150

How should I store the newer version premix pen? 150

Can you give me the summary for all the storage conditions? 151

I am taking premix two times a day, before breakfast and dinner. I forgot my morning dose. What should I do? 152

If I missed my pre-dinner dose, what can I do? 152

My sugar is high, can I have a sliding scale using premix insulin? 152

Which premix is the most affordable? 152

CHAPTER 13. MORE DETAILED PLANS FOR ADJUSTING INSULIN DOSAGE 153

I am using basal insulin and my sugar is 100 mg/dl. Should I give myself insulin or not? 153

What is my sugar target if I am taking basal insulin? 153

I am taking Toujeo, Lantus, Basaglar, or Tresiba as a basal insulin once a day at night, and my night time (bedtime) sugar is in the target, what is your general guideline? 155

I am taking Toujeo, Lantus, Basaglar, or Tresiba as a basal insulin once a day at night, and my night time (bedtime) sugar is above the target. What is your general guideline? 157

I am taking Toujeo, Lantus, Basaglar, or Tresiba as a basal insulin once a day at night, and my night time (bedtime) sugar is below the target. What is your general guideline? 159

I am taking pre-meal insulin, my morning sugar is too high. What can I do? 161

My pre-lunch sugar is too high. What can I do? 161

My pre-dinner sugar is too high. What can I do? 162

My morning sugar is too low. What can I do? 162

My pre-lunch sugar is too low. What can I do? 163

My pre-dinner sugar is too low. What can I do? 163

What are your general recommendations for low pre-meal sugar on that day? 163

What are your general recommendations for daily adjustment of pre-meal insulin? 164

CHAPTER 14. INSULIN USE FOR SHIFT-WORKERS 165

Why does shift work pose an extra challenge in using insulin? 165

What can I do to make my insulin use safer and more effective as a shift worker? 165

I am a shift worker with type 2 diabetes, and my doctor said I need to be on insulin. What is your recommendation? 166

I have type 1 diabetes and I am a shift worker. What is my best option? 167

I have type 1 diabetes and I am a shift worker and have to stay on shots. What is your recommendation? 168

CHAPTER 15. TRUCK DRIVERS AND INSULIN **169**

Can I be a truck driver or continue to be a truck driver if I have Type 2 diabetes and use insulin? 169

What is FMCSA Diabetes Waiver? 169

From a medical point of view, how do I prepare for the exemption application? 169

How will endocrinologists evaluate to assess your diabetes control? 170

What can I do if my endocrinologist is not willing to fill out the form? 171

What else can I do if I cannot get my endocrinologist on board? 172

I have type 2 diabetes, and I am a truck driver. What can I do as a truck driver to avoid insulin in the future? 172

CHAPTER 16. QUESTIONS ABOUT HIGH AND LOW BLOOD SUGAR LEVELS AND DEALING WITH STEROIDS **175**

What symptoms or signs might indicate low sugar? 175

What should I do if I feel my sugar is low? 175

How should I treat low sugar? 176

What should I do if my sugar is low and I do not feel it? 177

What should I do if I cannot feel when my sugar is low? 177

When should I use the glucagon shot my doctor prescribed for me?. 178

How should I use the glucagon shot? 178

When should I go to the hospital if I have low sugar? 179

What should I do to prevent hypoglycemia? 179

What medications might increase my chance of having low sugar? . 180

My morning sugar is always high. What can I do? 180

When do I need to check urine ketones? 182

What do I need to do if my ketones are positive? 183

What should I do if I have nausea and vomiting and I am unable to keep anything down?.. 183

What should I do if my sugar goes above 500 after a steroid shot? .. 183

I am on steroids. Do you have some general recommendations?...... 184

What should I do if my sugar goes over 500 and I am not taking steroids? 185

What are the common reasons for sugar to go over 500?................. 185

I am on an insulin pump. My sugar goes over 500. What should I do? 186

What should I do if for no reason my sugar goes over 500? 187

What should I do if my sugar is persistently higher than 250 and I do not feel well? 187

I started on a new batch of insulin, and now I cannot get my sugar down. What should I do?... 188

I am going to have colonoscopy or day-surgery. Should I take my insulin and how should I take it? 188

CHAPTER 17. FINAL WORDS-ALL ABOUT INSULIN 189

Why should I not be afraid of insulin?... 189

How can we reduce insulin use?.. 189

Anything else can I do to make my insulin use safer? 190

"Insulin is one of the greatest scientific discoveries, but using it is not a science; it is an art."

–Words of my patient

Chapter 1. General information about starting insulin

What basic information should I know before starting insulin injections?

- ➤ Learn why you need to be started on insulin.
- ➤ Learn the name and dosage of your insulin.
- ➤ Before you inject, you need to double check which insulin and at what dose, because insulin can be very dangerous. If you take the wrong type of insulin or the wrong dose, it can cause major problems with your blood sugar-either high or low- and even death.
- ➤ Always check the vial or pen to make sure the liquid is not clumped and not expired. Expiration dates are vary.
- ➤ Try your best to learn the basics of insulin: long-acting vs. short-acting, how soon it will start working, how long it will work, etc. If you are unsure ask your physician.
- ➤ Always check your sugar before injecting insulin.
- ➤ Always be prepared for low/high sugar. Learn the signs and symptoms of low and high sugar and how to manage them properly.
- ➤ Report to your treating physician if you have low sugars. This may require an urgent visit, especially if you have a low sugar episode which requires another person to help you correct your low sugar: we call this severe

hypoglycemia since you cannot correct the problem yourself. If you have loss of consciousness or seizure, or you can not correct your sugar yourself, you need to go to the ER immediately.

➢ Always prime your pen (remove air from the needle and pen or syringe), especially when your dose is less than 20 units. Put on needle and select 2 units, pointing to the air, inject to see the fluid from the needle. If you do not see any, you need to repeat the process. Sometimes if you have bad vision, you might not able to see it. In this case, I strongly recommend using pen, then 2 units of priming is definitely enough. Sometimes, you might have a bad needle, you need to change the needle too.

➢ If you are using a syringe, make sure you are injecting through a U100 syringe. You do not need to do any calculations; If you are using a pen, just use the pen at the prescribed dose. To illustrate the importance of this problem I will cite an example of an actual patient experience: the patient came to see me for low blood sugars shortly after administering the insulin dose. Upon further discussion, it became clear that the patient, was trying to do some sort of calculation rather than simply giving the prescribed dose. The net result was he gave himself **100 units** instead of **10 units** and this was the explanation for the recurrent hypoglycemia.

➢ If you are using a pen, make sure to remove the entire needle protector and look at the needle before you give the injection. Some of my patients have tried giving the insulin injection with the needle protector still on, causing there to be **no insulin administered** with the injection, which then causes increasing blood sugar.

➢ In case of an emergency, get a Medical Alert necklace, bracelet, or card identifying you as an insulin-requiring diabetic patient. It is also a good idea to carry your medication list with you, including your allergies.

Where can I inject?

- The abdomen, but at least one inch from the belly button. This is the most common area I asked my patient to start. The insulin absorption is most stable.
- The upper outer area of the arms.
- The top outer area of the thighs. Insulin usually is absorbed more slowly from this site, but if you exercise soon after injecting, then insulin will be absorbed faster from your legs.

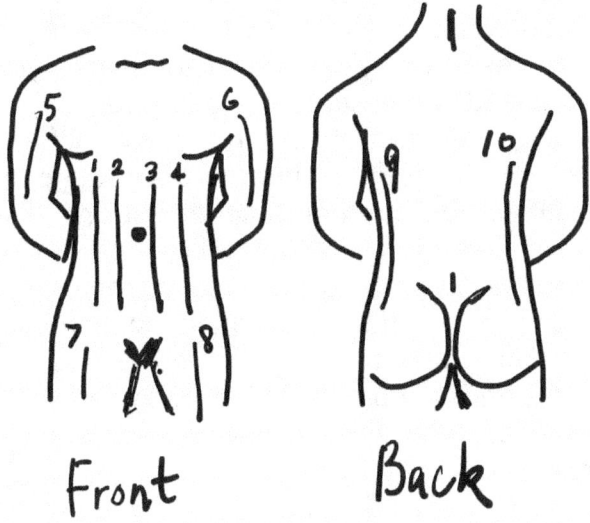

Front   Back

Figure. Picture I draw for my patients to illustrate where to do the injection. The lines are for rotating purpose. I ask my patients to inject both sides along the lines, and rotate these lines.

Which one is better? Pen or vial?

I like pens better, because you do not have to draw the insulin. They are much easier, especially for the elderly. Pens are also more convenient to use when you go out to eat. They can easily fit in your purse or pocket. However, pens are more expensive per unit.

Which needle is better?

Most needles do not cause any pain. I recommend to use the smallest needle possible. My patients have reported that Novofine Plus is very good.

What are the potential short-term adverse effects?

> Insulin significantly increases your risk for hypoglycemia.
> Allergic reactions: If you have severe rashes, breathing problems, sweating, or more severe reactions causing low blood pressure, shock, lip and /or tongue swelling or breathing difficulties (anaphylaxis, or angioedema), **you need to go to the ER immediately** and have a family member or friend notify your physician about what has happened. **Do not waste time trying to contact your doctor yourself as you need medical attention promptly.**
> Low potassium. Insulin drives potassium into the cells. Simply put insulin lowers the potassium in the blood as it encourages the potassium to move into your body's cells. This can cause significant problems including heart rhythm irregularities, muscle cramps, weakness and even excessive urination.
> Heart failure and fluid retention, especially if you are also taking medications such as Actos (chemical name pioglitazone) or Avandia (chemical name rosiglitazone). It is worth noting that this phenomenon is more likely in patients that are prone to edema (swelling) such as heart failure, patients with significant kidney problems, or liver disease- although these conditions do not necessarily need to be present for the edema to occur.

What are the potential long-term adverse effects of insulin?

➤ Weight gain is common with insulin. Please review other sections to learn how to mitigate this.

➤ Injection site lipohypertrophy– meaning induction of fat tissue -which has very limited blood supply. The net effect if you inject in such a site is that the insulin may not be absorbed into the bloodstream, and a high blood sugar can ensue. This could be related to repeated injury of the injection site and could be exacerbated by other chemicals in the insulin solution like phenol or its derivatives. Therefore, you are advised to use the lowest possible dose and **rotate your injection sites.** Your physician or diabetes educator will show you how to rotate your injection sites so that you minimize the chance of these problems occurring. Note that lipoatrophy can also occur, which could accelerate the speed at which insulin is absorbed, potentially resulting in low blood sugar.

➤ Insulin antibody formation. This antibody might cause your sugar to become unstable. You may not know this is happening; however, one clue to the presence of this problem is a significant change in your blood sugar control which you have difficulty explaining: unexpected high and low blood sugar may result in this setting and you need to notify your doctor about the change in your blood sugar control.

➤ Insulin can cause fluid retention leading to swelling.

What can I expect after I start insulin injection?

➤ It is not uncommon for people just starting on insulin-especially if they have had hyperglycemia for some time-to have the feeling that they are experiencing a low blood sugar; this perception may occur even when their sugar levels are normal - that is to say as measured on the home glucose monitor. With uncontrolled diabetes, your body has become used to high sugar levels, and when your sugars come back down to normal, your body reacts as if they were excessively low. This is why I recommend that patients start insulin at lower doses and gradually increase insulin doses with subsequent adjustments as advised by the treating physician. It took some time to develop the problem of high blood sugars and it is common sense to assume that adjusting to normalization of the blood sugar may require a bit of time as well. If you feel low blood sugar symptoms right after starting insulin, you can treat yourself as if you actually had low sugars. Please also talk to your doctor for further guidance.

➢ Blurred vision might occur when it was not previously noted. This occurs because your eyes need a certain pressure to maintain their shape to ensure that your vision is working properly. Sugars contribute to the eye pressure. When your sugar changes-especially rapidly and significantly, the shape of your eyes might change, resulting in problems with visual clarity or the ability of your eyes to focus on a given object. This needs to be understood by you for two reasons. First , do not panic if this occurs the vision will improve if initially blurred. Second, it is better to get an eye exam for example with an ophthalmologist when your eyes have accommodated to the new levels of your blood sugar. Again the change in vision is short lived so give it some time.

➢ If you have had retinopathy- a term meaning the presence of diabetic eye disease in the retina which is like the "film" of your eye- before starting insulin and your sugars have been poorly controlled, your retinopathy might get worse after your sugars suddenly become normal. Again, this should get better over time.

➢ Your neuropathy might get worse before getting better. The exact cause is still not clear. In general neuropathy which commonly causes symptoms of numbness tingling, burning of the lower extremities- especially the soles of the feet particularly at night- may get worse. It is important to understand that neuropathy may or may not improve with favorable changes in blood sugar profile.

Unfortunately, the reasons for this is not well understood. In contrast, retinopathy and nephropathy (kidney disease) tend to get better with improved glycemic control.

➤ The pain caused by insulin injections should be minimal. If you have severe pain, you need to talk to your doctor. Something may be wrong.

What if some insulin leaks back out of the injection site?

When insulin leaks back after injection, do not try to gauge the amount lost and replace it; you might run the risk of giving too much insulin and cause your blood sugar to fall too low. Record it in your logbook and take it into account if the next blood check is high. In the meantime, Here are a few things you can do to prevent this from happening with subsequent insulin injections:

➤ You can try to pinch the skin and then give the injection.

➤ After the injection, count to 10, and then stop pinching the skin, and finally at that moment, then remove your needle.

➤ Do not reuse the needle.

➤ Ask your doctor to prescribe smaller needles.

➤ If you are on a high dose, ask your doctor to prescribe more concentrated insulin. Examples of this category of insulins are as follows: Toujeo is three times more concentrated U-300; Tresiba has two versions of insulin: one type is usual U-100 insulin concentration and the other is 2x as concentrated U-200. Both Toujeo and Tresiba are long acting or basal insulins. Humalog- a short acting insulin- also has 2 different versions similar to Tresiba (U-100 and U200).

➤ If your insurance does not cover the more concentrated version, you can try to inject two doses. As examples, taking Levemir two times a day. or Lantus , or Basaglar two times a day, may be better than single daily dosing.

What should I do if there is bleeding or bruising at the injection site?

Sometimes the needle can hit a small blood vessel and cause bleeding and bruises. If this happens infrequently, you have nothing to worry about. But if it happens often, you need to talk to your doctor. You might have a bleeding disorder; you might need to change to smaller needles; your injection procedure may need to be improved and reviewed with a diabetic educator.

What should I do if I have injection site redness and itchiness?

You might have an allergic or nonallergic reaction to a noninsulin component in the insulin preparation. You might need to change to a different brand or formula. In rare cases, it may be an allergic reaction to insulin. You need to raise this issue with your doctor.

What happens if you accidentally inject too much insulin?

This depends on how well your sugars are controlled, how much you inject and what kind of insulin you are using. For fast-acting insulin, you can eat more depending on how much insulin you took, based on carbohydrate ratio or proportion to meal insulin. If you overdosed with long-acting insulin during the day, you can reduce your pre-meal fast-acting insulin proportionally if you are taking pre-meal insulin also, or eat more. Importantly, **you will need to monitor your sugar more closely for the next 16-24 hours.** If you overdosed with long-acting insulin at night, you need to eat some snacks and ask friends or family to wake you up every 2-4 hours to check your sugar. Taking a snack will depend upon the baseline status of your blood sugar control.

What happens if an air bubble was accidentally injected?

You do not need to worry about the bubble itself. However, if you are **not** getting a full dose of insulin, your sugars may go up. You do not have to add more insulin; you can just correct it with the next injection.

Can I reuse my needles or syringes?

It is not recommended to reuse needles; this can increase the risk of injection site infection or injury. The risk for injection site pain, bleeding, or bruising also increases.

It is also not recommended to reuse syringes because doing so increases the risk for infections.

Can I leave the needle on the pen (after I have already used this needle for a prior injection) to be used for new injection?

This is not recommended because it can decrease accuracy , leak insulin, and increase the risk for infection and injury.

I have type 2 diabetes, and I was recommended to start insulin. Does it mean I have to be on insulin forever?

Absolutely not! If your sugars get too high, it can cause something called "glucotoxicity" to the beta cells that secrete insulin. When insulin is used properly, it can reduce glucotoxicity and help to recover and preserve your beta cells. I have many patients who were initially started on insulin, but after lifestyle modifications through diet and exercise, **were able to get off insulin**. As a matter of fact, I have many patients who have been able to achieve diabetes remission, meaning they no longer require any diabetes medications.

I have type 2 diabetes, why should I start insulin?

Diabetes is a progressive disease. At the beginning of type 2 diabetes, there is already an insulin deficiency of 50%. As the disease progresses, insulin deficiency becomes more severe, especially with poor control of the blood sugars.

Research shows that insulin, if used early, can help your insulin-producing cells (beta cells) recover from glucotoxicity. This is good news because it means insulin **may** be stopped as sugar control improves.

What precautions must I take if I am using insulin and driving?

The major side effect for insulin is hypoglycemia. I have patients who sadly, were killed, or killed other people while driving because of hypoglycemia, so p**lease take this seriously.**

How to prepare:
1) Always wear a medical alert bracelet that says you have diabetes and that you are on insulin.
2) Have a diabetes kit with you at all times. The kit should include a glucometer, test strips, lancet, alcohol swabs, insulin, and glucose tablets. If you have severe hypoglycemia or history of loss of consciousness, I do not recommend to drive.
3) Check your sugars before you drive. The level should be above 100: if not take a snack and make sure sugar >100 prior to driving.
4) If possible, wear a sensor (continuous glucose monitor).
5) If you are driving long distances, check your blood sugar every 2 hours.
6) Stop and check your sugars if you feel symptoms of hypoglycemia (see hypoglycemia section).
7) Do not drive until your sugars have stabilized.
8) Alcohol taken shortly before driving can cause a sudden low blood sugar and should be avoided.
9) These steps may seem laborious, but your life, and the lives of others around you are in your hands.

Which type of insulin is best?

There is no single best type of insulin. Every type of insulin serves different purposes for different people, and depends on the circumstances.

What is long-acting insulin(basal insulin)?

Again, in this book, I use long-acting, slow-acting, basal insulin interchangeably. Long-acting insulin starts between one and two hours after injection and lasts at least 16-36 hours or longer. Here are the examples:

- Levemir (detemir)

- Lantus(glargine)

- Basaglar (glargine)

- Toujeo (glargine)

- Tresiba (degludec)

What is short-acting insulin (rapid-acting insulin, fast-acting insulin)?

In this book, I use short-acting, rapid-acting, fast-acting insulin, pre-meal insulin, prandial insulin interchangeably. When these insulins are used in insulin pump. Sometimes they also are referred to as bolus insulin.

It usually starts to act 10-30 minutes after injection, and lasts 2-6 hours. We usually use it before meals or for the sliding scale (correction scale).

Some doctors consider new insulin (Humalog, Novolog, Apidra) as rapid-acting and Humulin R and Novolin R as fast-acting insulin. However, they are all short-acting. You do not need to distinguish rapid-acting or fast-acting.

The FDA has just approved a new formula of Novolog called Fiasp rapid-acting insulin in September 2017. It can appear in the blood as soon as 2.5 minutes after injection, however the meaningful effect may not been faster. However, FDA approved it to be used immediately before the meal and 20 minutes within the meal.

Are there any other types of insulin?

Other types of insulin include:

- Intermediate-acting insulin: NPH N (Novolin N, Humulin N).

- Again, In this book, I use short-acting insulin, fast-acting insulin, and bolus insulin interchangeably; I use long-acting insulin, slow-acting insulin, and basal insulin interchangeably. However, it is important to note that NPH, an intermediate-acting insulin peaks, whereas basal insulins (Lantus, Levemir, Tresiba) do not peak, or have much less prominent peak.

- Premixed insulin: Premixed insulins combine specific amounts of intermediate-acting and fast-acting insulin in one bottle or insulin pen. Examples of these include Humalog mix 75/25, Humulin mix 70/30, Novolog mix 70/30, and Novolin mix 70/30.
- Combinations of long-acting (basal) insulin and GLP-1 agonist: Soliqua 100/33 is a combination of insulin glargine (Lantus) and the GLP-1 receptor agonist lixisenatide (Adlyxin in the US and Lyxumia in Europe). Another such combination is Xultophy 100/3.6. This is a combination of insulin Tresiba (degludec) and the GLP-1

agonist Victoza (liraglutide). These can only be used for type 2 diabetes.

- Inhaled insulin: Afrezza® is a rapid-acting (short-acting) inhaled insulin shown to improve glycemic control in adult patients with diabetes. This was approved by the FDA in 2014. It is a pre-meal insulin to be used with both type 1 and type 2 diabetes. In type 1 diabetes, Afrezza needs to be used with long-acting insulin.

Table 1. Generic/Brand names and basic characteristics for fast-acting/rapid-acting/short-acting insulins:

Type of Insulin & Brand Names	Onset	Peak	Duration	Role in Blood Sugar Management
Lispro (Humalog)	15-30 min.	30-90 min.	3-5 hours	Rapid-acting insulin covers insulin needs for meals eaten after the injection. This type of insulin is often used with long-acting insulin. This is also used for correction.
Aspart (Novolog)	15-20 min.	40-50 min.	3-5 hours	
Aspart/ Niacinamide (Fiasp)	10-15	30-40 min.	3-5 hours	
Glulisine (Apidra)	20-30 min.	30-90 min.	3-4 hours	
Regular (R) Humulin or Novolin	30 min. -1 hour	2-5 hours	5-8 hours	Short-acting insulin covers insulin needs for meals eaten within ½-1 hour

Table 2. Intermediate insulin

Type of insulin	Onset	Peak	Duration	Role in Blood Sugar Management
NPH (N) Novolin N, Humulin N	1-2 hours	4-12 hours	18-24 hours	Intermediate-acting insulin covers insulin needs for about half a day or overnight. This type of insulin is often combined with a rapid- or short-acting type.

Table 3. Long-acting/slow-acting/basal insulin

Type of Insulin & Brand Names	Onset	Peak	Duration	Role in Blood Sugar Management
Insulin glargine (Lantus)	1-1½ hours	No peak time. Insulin is delivered at a steady level.	20-24 hours	Long-acting insulin covers insulin needs for about one full day. This type is often combined with fasting-acting insulin, when needed,
Insulin glargine 3X (Toujeo)	1-2 hours	No peak; at steady level	24-36 hours	
Insulin degludec (Tresiba	1-2 hours	No peak; at steady level	36-48 hours	
Insulin detemir (Levemir)	1-2 hours	6-8 hours	Up to 24 hours	

Table 4. Brand names for premixed insulins

Type of Insulin & Brand Names	Onset	Peak	Duration	Role in Blood Sugar Management
Humulin 70/30	30 min.	2-4 hours	14-24 hours	These products are generally taken two or three times a day before mealtime. Humulin 50/50, Humalog 50/50 are being discontinued.
Novolin 70/30	30 min.	2-12 hours	Up to 24 hours	
Novolog 70/30	10-20 min.	1-4 hours	Up to 24 hours	
Humulin 50/50,	30 min.	2-5 hours	18-24 hours	
Humalog mix 75/25, Humalog 50/50	15 min.	30 min.-2½ hours	16-20 hours	
*Premixed insulins combine specific amounts of intermediate-acting and short-acting/rapid-acting insulin in one bottle or insulin pen. The numbers following the brand name indicate the percentage of each type of insulin.				

Soliqua 100/33, and Xultophy 100/3.6 are two long-acting insulin mixed with GLP-1 agonists. The two components do not have effect on each other in terms of drug onset peak, and lasting time.

Who can use inhaled insulin?

As indicated by the FDA, Afrezza can be used both in adult type 1 and type 2 diabetes patients. It should not be used if you are a smoker, have COPD, asthma, or other chronic lung diseases. I also recommend that you use other forms of insulin if you have a respiratory infection or have been diagnosed with lung cancer.

What should I do if I forget to take my long-acting insulin (basal insulin, slow-acting insulin)?

This depends on what you are taking and how often you are taking it.

❖ If you are taking Tresiba, you usually are asked to take it once a day in the morning or night (you can take it at any time of the day). If you forget one dose, you can take it as soon as possible. You can go back to the regular schedule of injections as long as your next regularly scheduled injection is at least 8 hours away. If your regularly scheduled injection is within 8 hours, you can give one shot as soon as possible, then give another shot after 12 hours, and then go back to your regular schedule.

❖ If you are using Basaglar, Toujeo, Lantus, or Levemir once a day and miss a dose, and you want to keep your original schedule. You have many ways to handle it, but it's more complicated. Here are my recommendations:

➤ If scheduled next dose >12 hours, give your full dose as soon as possible, and then give half of your usual dose for next usual dose and at usual scheduled time;
For example, if you are supposed to take Toujeo 24 units at 9 pm, and you forget this dose until 9 am the following day, you can give the Toujeo

19

dose in the morning. HOWEVER, for your next dose, use 1/2 of your usual dose at 9 pm same day. That means if typically you take Toujeo 24 units at 9 pm and you forget this dose, at 9 am the following morning take Toujeo 24 units. That night at 9 p m you need to cut Toujeo dose to 12 units (half of your morning Toujeo is still working) and continue the usual schedule and usual dose next day. This approach can be used for missed doses of Lantus (Basaglar as well), or Levemir if used once a day.

➤ If scheduled next dose >8 hours, but less than 12 hours, give your usual dose as soon as possible, and then give ⅓ of your usual dose for next dose; For example, if you are supposed to take Toujeo 24 units at 9 pm, and you forget this dose until noon the following day, you can give the Toujeo dose as soon as possible. HOWEVER, for your next dose, give a third of your usual dose at 9 pm same day. That means if typically you take Toujeo 24 units at 9 pm and you forget this dose, at noon the following day take Toujeo 24 units. That night at 9 p m you need to cut Toujeo dose to 8 units (two third of your noon Toujeo is still working) and continue the usual schedule and usual dose next day. This approach can be used for missed doses of Lantus (Basaglar as well), or Levemir if used once a day.

➤ If scheduled next dose <8 hours, give your dose as soon as possible. You skip the dose at regular scheduled time same day, and then back to usual schedule next day.
For example, if you are supposed to take Toujeo at 9 pm, and you forget this dose until 5 pm the following day, you can give the Toujeo dose as soon as possible. HOWEVER, for your next dose, you skip your usual dose at 9 pm same day. That

means if typically you take Toujeo 24 units at 9 pm and you forget this dose until next day 5 pm, at 5 pm you take your Toujeo. That night at 9 pm you skip a Toujeo dose and continue the usual schedule and usual dose next day. This approach can be used for missed doses of Lantus (Basaglar as well), or Levemir if used once a day.

❖ If you are taking Basaglar, Lantus or Levemir every 12 hours,

➤ If scheduled next dose > 6 hours, give you full dose as soon as possible, and then give 1/2 of your usual dose for next usual time; then back to usual dose and usual schedule.
➤ If scheduled next dose <6 hours, give your dose as soon as possible, then just miss your next scheduled dose. Afterwards, then you can go back to usual schedule for next dose.

❖ NPH every 12 hours, you can follow the same correction as above every 12 hour regimen. However, NPH has a much more pronounced peak. You need to check your sugar more often.

❖ If you are taking pre-mixed insulin, it is much more complicated. You should call your doctor for advice. If you have type 2 diabetes, you might just have to miss a dose and not use the catch-up dose. If you have type 1 diabetes, you need to give your insulin as soon as you can. For next time, it is usually okay to give the usual dose and usual time, but you have to monitor your sugar more closely, since type 1 diabetes prone to have high and low sugars.

What should I do if I accidentally inject short-acting insulin for long-acting insulin?

If you are taking both long-acting and short-acting insulins. Sometimes distinguishing long-acting and short-acting insulin can be confusing. I often get calls about what to do if a patient mixes up the long-acting and short-acting insulin. Therefore, before you inject, you need to make sure which insulin you are supposed to injection.

Here is what you need to do:

1. **Do not panic.**

2. Depending on your sugar level and insulin sensitivity, your reaction to this situation will be different for different people.

3. Usually, the dose for long-acting is three times as much as short-acting, and short-acting works faster. Therefore, the problem at hand is avoiding low blood sugar from occurring.

4. So, I recommend eating a "full meal" (as much as carbs in your usual meal) and then rechecking your blood sugar 2 hours later and once again another 2 hours later. (meaning 4 hours from the original injection). **The goal is to avoid your blood sugar from dropping to below 70**- and this is especially true if you have underlying kidney disease or heart disease, or history of stroke. If the blood sugar at 2 hours and 4 hours sometimes 6 hours after the initial "episode" is fine (>130), go to bed and resume your usual insulin regimen the following morning. Otherwise, eat another snack, It is very important to notify your spouse for example or even call a friend to check in on you 2-6 hours after the original mistaken dose of insulin was taken.

5. If you have type 1 diabetes, it is better to give long acting insulin if you have not been given it yet. As a precaution, inject half of your usual dose 2 hours later if your sugar is going up (>130). If you have type 2 diabetes, it is not so crucial to give or not to give the long acting. You can give the half dose as type 1 diabetes, or just omit long acting for one day. You can always adjust your short-acting for next meal.

6. If you are in a situation in which you do not have a meal to eat, you can eat the same carbs as your usual meal and do the insulin as above. Check your sugar every 1-2 hours to make sure you are not developing low sugar in next 4-6 hours. If you develop low sugar, treat accordingly. If going up, you are okay.

7. If you are alone and you do not have anything to eat, and you cannot check your sugar, call your friend or family to help, otherwise, you have to call 911 as soon as possible.

What should I do if I accidentally inject long-acting insulin (slow-acting, basal insulin) for short-acting insulin (fast-acting, rapid-acting insulin)?

It is slightly more challenging in this case, but there is **no need to panic.** Actually, the chances of your developing low sugar is much lower compared to the mistake of injecting short-acting for long-acting because the short-acting dose and the long-acting doses are different. Usually the short-acting dose is a third of long-acting. You inject long-acting. They act differently (you can get more details about this by consulting the tables provided above outlining duration of action, peak of the various insulins etc.). Here are a few scenarios:

Shunzhong Shawn Bao, MD

Scenario 1: You usually injection of both short-acting and long-acting in the mooring, and you injected long-acting for short-acting insulin in the morning.

1. As we discussed above, your usual short-acting dose is lower than long-acting. Now you injected long-acting for short-acting, therefore you have underdoes yourself for long acting. This is easy. You can just supplement the rest long-acting.
2. For example, you are supposed to take Lantus 30 units in the morning and 10 units of Humalog before each meal. Now you injected Lantus for 10 units. You inject Lantus thought as Humalog. Now you have not injected your short-acting yet, so give it. Also you have not given enough long-acting Lantus. You need to give the difference of 20 units more (30 units-10 units).

Scenario 2: You usually inject long-acting at night, and now you give your long-acting as short-acting before breakfast.

1. In this case, you gave yourself extra long-acting, but have not given short-acting yet.
2. I recommend you go ahead to give your usual short-acting insulin but reducing it by 25% or half of short-acting for the rest of the day if you are prone to have low sugars.
3. At the same night, if you sugar is >130, you can give the full dose of your long-acting insulin. If not, you can eat some snack and then given half of your usual dose depending your propensity to have low sugar.
4. For example, you are taking Lantus 36 units at night and 12 units of Humalog before each meal. In the morning you injected Lantus 12 units. You can go ahead to inject 6-9 units (reduced by 25-50%) short-acting for your meal for the rest of the day. At night, if your sugar is above 130 you can give the full dose of Lantus, otherwise eat some snack and raise your sugar to above to 130, and then give 18 units if you are prone to have low sugar,

otherwise give 30 units Lantus (36-12/2). 36 units is your regular dose. 12/2 is half of the Lantus which is still in your system.

Scenario 3. You usual injection of long-acting in the morning. You gave yourself correct dose in the morning but you made mistake at lunch. You inject long-acting as short acting before lunch.

1. I recommend you reduce your short-acting by 25% for the rest of the day.
2. For the long-acting next morning, I also recommend by 25% of the injected dose by mistake.
3. Second day, you take your normal short-acting dose.
4. For example, you take 36 Lantus in the morning, and 12 units of Humalog before each meal. In the morning you inject the right long-acting and short-acting insulin. Before lunch you grab a wrong insulin pen. You injected yourself 12 units of Lantus. You should have injected yourself 12 units of Humalog. I recommend you go ahead to give yourself 9 units of Humalog (reduced by 25% of 12) for lunch. Then before dinner, you also give 9 units. Second day morning, when you get ready to give Lantus, If your sugar above 100, you can give your full dose of Lantus and everything back to usual. If your sugar above 70 but less than 100, I recommend to reduce your Lantus by 3 units (25% of 12). This means you should take Lantus 33 units (36-3).

Scenatio 4. You usual injection of long-acting is at bedtime. You inject your long-acting as short-acting before dinner by mistake.

1. In this case, I would recommend to go ahead to give your short acting normal dose or reduce it by 10% if you prone to have low sugar. I also recommend you continue to give yourself the long-acting insulin at your usual time but

     reducing the amount which is injected by mistake before dinner.

2. For example, if you usually give Lantus 36 units at bed time, and give 12 units of Humalog before each meal. You made mistake by giving Lantus 12 units before dinner. I recommend you continue to give Humalog 12 units or give 10 units if you prone to have low sugar. At bed time, you can give Lantus 24 units (36 units- 12 units). 36 units is your regular dose of Lantus; 12 is the dose you injected before meal by mistake.

Scenario 5. You usual injection of long-acting is at bedtime. You injected long-acting as short-acting before Lunch.

1. In this case, I recommend to inject short-acting but reducing by 10-20% for lunch and dinner. At night, you can continue to give long-acting, but reduce it by 25% of the injected dose by mistake at noon.
2. For example, if you are taking Lantus 36 units at bedtime, and taking Humalog 12 units before each meal. You injected Lantus 12 units before lunch as Humalog. I recommend to continue to give Humalog 9 units (reduced by 25% from 12 units usual dose) for lunch and dinner. At bedtime, I recommend you to give 27 units of Lantus as long-acting insulin (36 units – 9 units). 36 units is your usual long-acting dose; 9 units is the 75% of short-acting.

If you are prone to having low sugar (hypoglycemia) and your next meal is 5-6 hours away, you might need to check your sugar in 4 hours to make sure your sugar is not low.

If you have a CGM, then you can just set up your threshold, if you develop low sugar then treat accordingly. Again, I recommend everybody on insulin get on a CGM if possible.

What should I do if I accidentally inject myself with long-acting as short-acting and short-acting as long-acting?

Things happen. There is no need to panic.

If happened at breakfast time:

Some patients have both long-acting and short-acting insulin shots at the same time in the morning, which is no problem. Normally, the long-acting dose is three times as much as the short-acting dose, so you have given yourself three times the short-acting dose and one-third of the normal long-acting dose.

In the morning, your sugar may go down because you have too much short-acting insulin (usually 3 times as much). Therefore, you need to eat more breakfast (2-3 times more carbs). For afternoon and dinner time and second day morning, your sugar might go up since you have given only ⅓ of your long acting. However, you can just give sliding scale or correction dose using short-acting.

If this happens at supper time:

Well, this is why, I do not ask my patients to give long acting at supper time, but at bedtime to avoid this kind of mistake. Again, you can give your long-acting at supper time instead of bedtime, but this kind mistake can occur if you do that.

As we discussed above, since you gave yourself too much short-acting, you need to eat 2-3 times more carbs. And definitely need to check your sugar at bedtime to make sure it is not low.

Shunzhong Shawn Bao, MD

Check your sugar one more time between bedtime and early morning to make sure your sugar is not too low or high. It is very important to alert your spouse, loved ones or friend about this mistake, so they can alert you to check your sugar. If you follow this schedule, your sugar may be elevated slightly, which is good in this case. You can just give short-acting per correction scale or sliding scale. After 24 hours, go back to your regular schedule.

I was prescribed basal insulin two times a day, and the morning dose is so much more than night dose. I injected the morning dose at night. What should I do?

It depends how much you overdose and how your body responds to insulin. As we discussed earlier, **the risk in this circumstance is the occurrence of hypoglycemia or low blood sugar**. You need to closely monitor your sugar every 2-4 hours depending on how much you overdosed and how sensitive you are to insulin. In general if during this monitoring period, if your blood sugar goes below 100 you should eat a snack with carbs, and again closely monitor your sugar for at least 12 hours.

I recommend that you miss your morning dose the next day if your sugar is not too high, and get back to your schedule at night with the usual night dose. However, if your morning is above 100 and you might be able to resume your regular schedule. Mistakes happen. Insulin-especially injecting too much insulin at the wrong time, can be dangerous. Please be careful before injecting.

When I prescribe insulin, especially the first time, I always give detailed instruction, but there is so much to learn and so much information about it. It is impossible to write down everything for my patients. This is one of the reasons I wrote this book.

28

Why is pre-mixed insulin not optimal for type 1 diabetes?

Currently, we have analog pre-mixed insulin and regular fast-acting insulin pre-mixed.

For Humalog, we have a Humalog mix with NPH 50 / 50 (Humalog 50% and NPH 50%-going to be discontinued); we also have Humalog mix with NPH 75 / 25 (NPH 75% and Humalog 25%).

For Novolog mix with NPH 70 / 30 (NPH 70% and Novolog 30%).

For regular fast-acting insulin, we have NPH mixed with Humulin R or Novolin R 70/30 (70% NPH and 30% of regular insulin).

The benefit of pre-mixed is that only one shot is required for both fast-acting and intermediate-acting insulin (as supposed to two shots should the two insulins be injected separately).

The regular pre-mixed insulin is more affordable (Novolin 70/30 cost $26 for 1000 units at Wal-Mart or Sam's club pharmacy).

Disadvantages of pre-mixed insulin:

1. The ratio for fast-acting and intermediate-acting is fixed. You cannot change it as needed. This means for example, suppose your fasting blood sugar is high. Normally you would increase the amount of fasting insulin that you take in the same day or increase the intermediate insulin the previous night. In the premixed insulin, increasing the fast-acting insulin also means increasing the intermediate-acting insulin (which you may

not want to do). So, my opinion is that there is a price to be paid for the lack of dose flexibility. On the other hand, mixing insulin in the same syringe is not easy especially for people with arthritis or bad vision. The premixed insulin simplifies the process which may be helpful for individuals who have these problems.

2. Pre-mixed insulin is not easy to adjust. It is difficult to give a sliding scale or correction scale.

3. Pre-mixed insulin varies widely and needs to be mixed very well before usage.

Why are some insulins clear and other insulins cloudy?

Any insulin with NPH is cloudy. These are Novolin N, Humulin N, and any pre-mixed insulin.

How should I store insulin?

1. For unused insulin vials or pens, they should be stored in a refrigerator and never frozen. They should not be stored too close to the frozen compartment either. They can be stored until the expiration date on the vials or pens.

2. For a used vial, you can store at room temperature or in the refrigerator. Either way, it does not affect its potency. However, if you store it in the refrigerator, allow it to warm up to room temperature before giving the injection. This reduces irritation at the injection site.

3. If you start to use the vial, **the storage life ranges from seven days to one month depending on the brand. Please check the product package.**

4. For pens, after you start using them, **do not put them back into the refrigerator. Keep them at room temperature**. The following list details common brand storage life:

- Humalog U100 or U200 (28 days)
- Humulin N (14 days); Humalog mix 75/25 (10 days)
- Humalog mix 50/50 (10 days)
- Humulin mix 75/25 (10 days)
- Novolin R (28 days)
- Novolin N (14 days)
- Novolin 70/30 (10 days)
- Novolog (28 days), Fiasp (28 days)
- Toujeo (28 days)
- Tresiba (8 weeks)
- Lantus/Basaglar (28 days)

I do not have a good memory. I think I gave myself a shot a minute ago, but I am not sure if I did or did not. Is there anything I can do?

Insulin can be very dangerous. If this is the case for you, I would recommend that you discuss with your prescribing doctor if it is possible to avoid insulin in your regimen if you have type 2 diabetes. We have lots of other very effective regimens nowadays.

If you must use insulin, timer caps are available for your insulin pen. Every time you put on the cap, it starts a timer, so that you can see the last time you used the pen. This prevents you from injecting yourself twice. The timer cap is called a Timsulin smart pen cap. You can Google it or buy it from Kmart.

What else do I need to remember when I do an injection?

1. Only use injection sites that are smooth, with no signs of infection, bumps, or scars.

2. Always rotate the injection site.

3. If you take long-acting insulin, you can inject it on your thigh at night, because you will not be active. Movement and exercise can affect insulin absorption, so you need to be as consistent as possible.

4. Some patients use rotation tattoos, because it helps them keep track of injection sites.

If I have type 2 diabetes, what can I do to prevent weight gain with insulin use?

Insulin is an anabolic hormone, meaning that it helps synthesize the building blocks of your body and in this manner though not the intention insulin commonly causes weight gain. Insulin also can cause fluid retention (edema) which can also cause weight gain in the form of "water weight." Therefore, most patients on insulin gain weight. But if you take the following measures, you reduce the chances of gaining weight.

1. Try not to eat snacks while you are on insulin. Many doctors will ask you to eat snacks to prevent low sugar, but this is wrong. Eating more snacks will cause you to have a higher chance of having low sugar, because when you check your sugar, it will always be high. If your sugar is always high, your doctor will increase your insulin dose, because your sugar is not controlled, and you will gain more weight. I have detailed snack recommendation on snacks in my other book <<Diabetes Questions and Answers: More Than 400 Diabetes Frequently Asked Question>>.

2. Try to use the lowest dose possible for type 2 diabetes. Type 1 diabetes is more complicated. You need to talk to your doctor specifically about this issue.

3. Focus on lifestyle changes (see details in my other book- <<Diabetes Questions And Answers: More Than 400 Diabetes Frequently Asked Questions>>).

4. I recommend that you do some sort of exercise before each meal (a short walk may be reasonable for example), which will increase your insulin sensitivity, This will in most cases mean that you need to reduce the insulin dose for that meal. *Your doctor may help you with these adjustments*.

5. Cut down fatty meal intake, some meats have so much fat. Fat decreases your insulin sensitivity, and your dose will need to be increased.

6. Cut down on carbohydrates (carbs). **For type 1 diabetes, you cannot eat a "zero"** carbohydrate diet. This might cause severe ketosis and can be dangerous (the breakdown product of fat are substances called ketone bodies).

7. Ask your doctor if you qualify for use of insulin in combination with some newer diabetes medications which may curb your appetite and help you lose weight. These are the medications: GLP-1 agonists like Byetta, Bydureon, Trulicity, Tanzeum (discontinued), and Victoza all of which may decrease appetite; or SGLT2 antagonists (a different class or group of medication that work differently from the GLP-1class) like Farxiga, Invokana, and Jardiance. Acarbose, another type of blood sugar lowering medication, slows down the speed

by which sugars get into your bloodstream; this may prevent weight gain.

8. Ask your doctor to review your medication list to see if you can get off medications that cause weight gain.

Can you tell me more about basal and bolus regimen?

Usually, you are prescribed two kinds of insulin, long-acting and short-acting. The long-acting insulins (Lantus, Basaglar, Toujeo, Levemir, Tresiba) serve as basal insulin to be taken once or twice a day. Therefore, in discussion, we consider long-acting insulin, basal insulin, and slow-acting insulin interchangeably; we consider short-acting insulin, fast-acting insulin, premeal insulin, interchangeably. These are the "prandial" or mealtime insulins. When we give for the meal, we can also call it a "bolus" insulin especially associated with insulin pump.

The basal insulin is used to control fasting sugar and sugar between meals. We usually adjust your basal insulin based on fasting sugar for long term. I also recommend you occasionally adjust your daily dose based on night time sugar. If you have to change your basal insulin very often, you need to talk to your doctor to make sure you are on a right basal dose of insulin or something else needs to be changed.

The fast-acting insulin (Fiasp, Novolog, Humalog, Apidra, Humulin R and Novolin R-note the R or regular insulins are slower than the " log" insulins or apidra) are taken before each meal. These are the bolus insulins. They are for meals. You need to adjust your fast-acting insulin based on your post meal sugar or next premeal sugar (for example, we can adjust your lunch time dose based on 2 hours after lunch sugar or just based on pre-dinner sugar). You can adjust both long-acting and short-acting insulins. Usually, we recommend adjusting fast-acting insulin (bolus) more often than the long-acting insulin (basal).

If your premeal insulin dose is fixed or scheduled, you also call it fixed dose or scheduled dose regimen.

Do you have general tips on how to use fixed or scheduled dose insulin regimen?

For most type 2 diabetes, you might be prescribed to give certain fixed dose of insulin before you eat. We call this fixed or scheduled dose insulin regimen. For most type 1 diabetes, and some type 2 diabetes, premeal insulin dosing is based on the carb you plan to consume. We do not have an official name for this regimen yet. Let us call it variable dose regimen based on insulin carb ratio.

These are general insulin injection recommendations for fixed or scheduled doses (for example a patient that routinely takes Humalog 10 units at breakfast and does this regardless of the amount of carbohydrate he or she is eating). Maintain a routine of eating three meals every day and be as consistent as possible with the amount of carbohydrates in each meal as well as controlling your portion sizes. Non-starch vegetables do not require portion control. Exercise helps you burn calories, especially carbohydrates. A 20-30 minute walk after or before a meal is a good idea! Keep a written record of meals, sugar numbers, etc.! You might need to reduce your pre-meal insulin if you plan to exercise before or after the meal (see the exercise section in my other book -<<Diabetes Questions And Answers: More Than 400 Diabetes Frequently Asked Questions>>).

Other important tips:

1. Make sure to give yourself short-acting insulin 5-15 minutes before you eat. (Novolog and Fiasp closer to 5 minutes and Humalog closer to 15 minutes); for Novolin R or Humulin R should be given 20-30 minutes before you eat.

2. If you do not know how much you are going to eat. You can give a small dose (a third) before you eat and supplement the rest as soon as you finish eating. Think about this Novolog and maybe even Humalog given after the meal allowing determination of how much insulin to take based what you did or did not eat. If you are somebody who has appetite and stomach issues, and routinely are not sure how much you are going to eat. The new insulin Fisap may be better for you, because it has been reported to work faster. It is FDA licensed to give within 20 mins of eating as meal insulin.

3. If you eat out, always give insulin after you see your food, since you never know how much and when you will be served. My point is if you take your insulin when you order your meal and if it is served later, you may be setting yourself up for a low blood sugar.

4. Check your sugar before you give short-acting insulin. You can adjust your dose based on your sugar level. Keep your correcting/sliding scale handy, so you can adjust your insulin doses.

5. You can adjust your premeal short-acting insulin based on what and how much you eat, and your expected post-meal activity.

6. For example, if you plan to eat some chicken spinach salad, and there are no added carbs, you do not have to take premeal fixed dose insulin. If your sugar is high, continue to give the correction dose based on the sliding scale.

7. For example, if you plan to eat half of the amount of your usual meal, you should take half of the amount of your fixed premeal dose insulin.

8. For example, if you do not eat, do not give your usual premeal insulin except for sliding scale.

We call it fixed dose and ask you to take a certain amount of insulin before you eat, however, you still need to adjust your insulin dose based on how much you eat, what you eat, and your expected unusual activity after meal.

Long-acting insulins: Lantus, Basaglar, Toujeo, Levemir, Tresiba are to be injected at the same time every day (usually morning or at bedtime). Tresiba can be injected as a "catch up"—I recommend that you stick to the schedule.

ROTATE injection sites as instructed!

Physical activity lowers your blood sugar. Check your blood sugar before engaging in strenuous physical activities. Intense exercise will decrease your sugar faster. You need to be more vigilant when you are engaging in a very strenuous exercise.

You must establish a meal routine (three meals daily or four meals daily) and remain consistent in the amount of carbohydrates as well as controlling your portion sizes. If you would like to eat three meals plus one snack, that is fine. Talk to your doctor, so your regimen can be changed accordingly.

Insulin is a treatment, not a cure! DO NOT RELY ON INSULIN ALONE! Healthy eating, physical activity, keeping a record, and testing are key.

DO NOT STOP taking insulin without consulting your doctor and/or diabetes educator.

Check your sugar before you drive, and always keep some sugar or snacks in your car or purse in case of emergency.

Typically before you drive, a blood sugar of 100 or higher is desirable; certainly do not drive if your blood sugar is below 70.

What is a sliding scale? How do I use it?

The sliding scale is called a correction scale. You usually take fast-acting insulin to correct high sugar. The idea is to get your sugar down by injecting fast-acting insulin based on your "usual dose of premeal insulin" with the addition of sliding scale or extra insulin because the blood sugar is higher. Sliding scale can also be applied to bedtime blood sugars that are higher than they should be even though normally you would not take a "scheduled" dose of fast-acting insulin at this time.

Different patients need different scales. And at different times of the day, you may need a different scale. Certainly with different disease statuses, you need different scales. You need to discuss with your doctor which correction scale you need to use. I usually print a scale for my patients.

Can you give me some examples of the sliding scale (correction scale)?

Again, the corrective insulin for a higher blood sugar should only be done with fast-acting insulin. Although at higher sugar levels, insulin does not work as efficiently as at lower levels of sugar, The following two ways are most commonly used.

> ➤ Use a simple calculation. Let us say, if your doctor determines that 1 unit insulin can drop 40 mg/dl sugar (Insulin sensitivity factor). You can use the following formula to decide how much insulin you need:

Insulin units you need

=(Current sugar-target sugar)/insulin sensitivity factor

For example, if you current sugar is 200 mg/dl, and your insulin sensitivity factor is 40, and your sugar target is 120 mg/dl, then your "corrective insulin" dose is 2 units

Insulin needed=(200-120)/40= 2 units

Use pre-calculated charts to help you so you do not need to calculate and remember those numbers. For simplification, I will give the following examples. You may have a different scale. Your doctor and you need to decide which scale to use. Sometimes, you might use a different scale during the day or night.

Again, you cannot arbitrarily pick a scale to use. You need to discuss these matters with your physician to arrive at a sliding scale that works best for you. At any time, if you have concerns, you need to consult your physician. You need to call your physician, if your sugar is out of range or persistently high or low.

For 1 unit of insulin to correct sugar 10 mg/dl, but if used at night, you might want to reduce by 2 units

- For sugar 70-100, no added insulin
- For sugar 101-120, add 2 units
- For sugar 121-140, add 4 units
- For sugar 141-160, add 6 units
- For sugar 161-180, add 8 units
- For sugar 181-200, add 10 units
- For sugar 201-220, add 12 units
- For sugar 221-240, add 14 units
- For sugar 241-260, add 16 units
- For sugar 261-280, add 18 units
- For sugar 281-300, add 20 units
- For sugar 301-320, add 22 units
- For sugar 321-340, add 24 units
- For sugar 341-360, add 26 units
- For sugar 361-380, add 28 units
- For sugar 381-400, add 30 units
- For sugar>401 add 35 units

For 1 unit of insulin to correct sugar 20 mg/dl, but if used at night, you might want to reduce by 2 units

- For sugar 70-100, no added insulin
- For sugar 101-120, add 1 unit
- For sugar 121-140, add 2 units
- For sugar 141-160, add 3 units
- For sugar 161-180, add 4 units
- For sugar 181-200, add 5 units
- For sugar 201-220, add 6 units
- For sugar 221-240, add 7 units
- For sugar 241-260, add 8 units
- For sugar 261-280, add 9 units
- For sugar 281-300, add 10 units
- For sugar 301-320, add 11 units
- For sugar 321-340, add 12 units
- For sugar 341-360, add 13 units
- For sugar 361-380, add 14 units
- For sugar 381-400, add 15 units
- For sugar>401, add 17 units

For 1 unit of insulin to correct 30 mg/dl, but if used at night, you might want to reduce by 1 unit

- For sugar 70-100, no added insulin
- For sugar 101-130, add 1 unit
- For sugar 131-160, add 2 units
- For sugar 161-190, add 3 units
- For sugar 191-220, add 4 units
- For sugar 221-250, add 5 units
- For sugar 251-280, add 6 units
- For sugar 281-310, add 7 units
- For sugar 311-340, add 8 units
- For sugar 341-370, add 9 units
- For sugar 371-400, add 10 units
- For sugar >401, add 12 units.

For 1 unit of insulin to correct 40 mg/dl of sugar, if used at night, you might want to reduce by 1 unit

- For sugar 70-120, no added insulin
- For sugar 121-160, add 1 unit
- For sugar 161-200, add 2 units
- For sugar 201-240, add 3 units
- For sugar 241-280, add 4 units
- For sugar 281-320, add 5 units
- For sugar 321-360, add 6 units
- For sugar 361-400, add 7 units
- For sugar>401, add 10 units

For 1 units of insulin to correct 50 mg/dl of sugar, if used at night, you might want to reduce by 1-2 units

- For sugar 70-130, no added insulin
- For sugar 131-180, add 1 unit
- For sugar 181-220, add 2 units
- For sugar 221-270, add 3 units
- For sugar 271-320, add 4 units
- For sugar 321-370, add 5 units
- For sugar 371-420, add 6 units
- For sugar >421, add 8 units

For 1 units of insulin to correct 60 mg/dl of sugar, but if used at night, you might want to reduce by 1-2 units

- For sugar 70-140, no added insulin
- For sugar 141-200, add 1 unit
- For sugar 201-260, add 2 unit
- For sugar 261-320, add 3 units
- For sugar 321-380, add 4 units
- For sugar 381-440, add 5 units
- For sugar >441, add 7 units

For 1 units of insulin to correct 80 mg/dl of sugar, but if used at night, you might want to reduce by 1-2 units

- For sugar 70-150, no added insulin
- For sugar 151-230, add 1 unit
- For sugar 231-310, add 2 units
- For sugar 311-390, add 3 units
- For sugar 391-450, add 4 units
- For sugar> 451, add 5 units

For 1 units of insulin to correct 90 mg/dl of sugar, but if used at night, you might want to reduce by 1-2 units

- For sugar 70-160, no added insulin
- For sugar 161-250, add 1 unit
- For sugar 251-340, add 2 unit
- For sugar 341-430, add 3 units
- For sugar >431, add 4 units

For 1 units of insulin to correct 100 mg/dl of sugar, but if used at night, you might want to reduce by 1-2 units

- For sugar 70-180, no added insulin
- For sugar 181-280, add 1 unit
- For sugar 281-380, add 2 units
- For sugar 381-450, add 3 units
- For sugar >451, add 4 units

If at any time, your sugar is out of range, you need to let your doctor know. The fact that I provided so many different sliding scales illustrates how different diabetic patients have different requirements of insulin to bring a high blood sugar down to acceptable levels.

I have type 1 diabetes. Do you have general recommendations about how to adjust long-acting insulin?

Life is complicated, and type 1 diabetes and insulin can make your life even more complicated. These are my general recommendations, you certainly need to speak to your doctor about your specifics.

1. If you are giving long-acting insulin in the morning, and your sugar is >80 in the morning, and if you are very healthy and do not get low sugar easily, you can give a full dose of long-acting insulin. If your sugar is below 60, then you might need to eat something first. If your sugar is between 60 and 80, you can give half of your long-acting insulin dose. It is important that you seek more specific advice from your doctor for your particular situation.

2. If you are giving your long-acting insulin at night and if your sugar is >130 at bedtime, you can give the full dose. If your sugar is between 100 and 130, you might need to cut down your night time long-acting insulin by half or 1/3. If your sugar is below 100, then you might need to eat a small snack and then give a half dose of long-acting insulin. This is tricky. You also need to learn from your experience. The recommendation here is just a starting point for you.

3. If you have frequently high or low sugar, you need to talk to your doctor. Your insulin regimen might need to be adjusted.

I have type 2 diabetes. Do you have a general recommendation about how to adjust long-acting insulin?

If you are relatively healthy, and if you do not experience hypoglycemia easily, you can follow the recommendations I gave for type 1 diabetes above.

If you have multiple comorbidities (heart disease, kidney disease or liver disease) or are very fragile, I would raise your sugar slightly. If your bedtime sugar is above 160, you can give the full dose. If it is between 130 and 160, you can consider half of the dose. If it is below 130, then you can omit the dose completely.

My previous doctor recommended I not change my basal insulin dose. What is your rationale behind adjusting my basal insulin dose?

As we discussed before, basal insulin is used to control fasting sugar. We usually adjust the dose based on the fasting sugar level. Most doctors believe that fasting sugar is most determined by insulin sensitivity and they believe sensitivity does not change much. The truth is that fasting sugar also is determined by your night time sugar level, your diet, emotion status and other things.

I recommend adjusting basal insulin dose for the following reasons:

1. It is safer if you check your blood sugar before you give insulin. I give my patients parameters for more precise insulin dosing; as a part of the guidelines, my patients are required to check their blood sugar more often, reducing the risk of hypoglycemia.
2. Some patients have acute changes in their circumstances, such as dehydration, strenuous exercise, special events with distinctive food requirements, etc. that change their need for insulin.
3. For patients who would normally eat a snack when their blood sugars are borderline, I would recommend that they reduce or omit the insulin (type 1 diabetes cannot skip insulin) instead of eating an additional snack. This has the added benefit of weight loss.

Is there an app to help me calculate my insulin dosage?

When we use apps or machines, we tend to trust the apps or machine more than our own instincts. If you take an overdose of insulin, it could harm you or even worse. Therefore, unless your doctor is familiar with the particular app, I do not recommend that you use it. I have a patient who uses an old insulin pump to calculate his insulin dosage. I put in all the settings, and he uses it to calculate his bolus. This is okay with me.

What should I do with those needles and sharps?

You know you should not throw away your sharps into the regular trash bin, but you might not know what to do with them. In America, every community has a Community Sharps Collection Program. The Community Sharps Collection Program usually provides a free container. If you do not know of a program, you can ask your doctor.

You can go to this website (http://www.safeneedledisposal.org/) to locate the nearest sharp disposal site. You can also call 1-800-643-1643 to find a location.

If your community does not have one, there are also sharp disposal mail programs. You can try Pureway Sharps Disposal System (pureway.com), GRP Sharps Disposal (sharpsdisposal.com), or Sharps Compliance (sharpsinc.com).

You can also contact your local health department for further information.

What is a proposed target of sugar and A1c?

Again, your target should be individualized. Your doctor and you should sit down and talk about it. This is certainly the approach recommended by the American Diabetes Association and other professional associations. Your diabetic regimen could and should be altered due to changing situations. Lots of factors affect your target. Your tendency to have low sugar arguably most important factor especially if you have heart disease, history of stroke or kidney or liver diseases (see below). These "comorbidities" (conditions) intensify the negative consequences of a low blood sugar.

Less stringent or more stringent targets based on:

> ➢ Hypoglycemia tendency
> ➢ Diabetes duration
> ➢ Age
> ➢ Microvascular or macrovascular complications (like kidney failure, cardiovascular disease)
> ➢ CVD (cardiovascular disease) risk factors
> ➢ Comorbidities (again like kidney failure, history of heart stents, bypass surgery)
> ➢ Financial means
> ➢ Self-motivation
> ➢ Social support (family, friends, or family members with or without diabetes themselves)
> ➢ Cognitive status
> ➢ And many other factors

If you are young with short duration of the disease, and do not easily experience low sugars and are motivated to have good blood sugar control, have good financial means, and social support, I recommend striving to get your sugar and A1c as normal as possible. I have had lots of patients who achieve this goal of normality and several of them have even experienced remission. This is only true of type 2 diabetes.

Normal Target:

➢ Fasting and before meals: 70-100 mg/dl
➢ 2 hour after meal: <140 mg/dl
➢ A1c target <5.5%

If you are very healthy except for diabetes and have the financial means, you also need to be very motivated. However, you are not able to get "normal". Given this context, it is reasonable that you choose "very tight control target". Reaching normal A1C values, for example, requires a great deal of effort; and maintaining this level of control is in many ways a " full time job." People are different and have different life circumstances and different capabilities; it is logical therefore that their A1C goals should be different.

Very Tight Control Target:

➢ Fasting and before meals: 70-110 mg/dl
➢ 2 hours after meal <140 mg/dl
➢ A1c of 6.0%

For most patients, you can reach the following target-"tight control target", This is the recommendation from American Association of Clinical Endocrinologist (AACE) for most patients.

Tight Control Target:

➢ Fasting and before meals: 70-120 mg/dl
➢ 2 hours after meal <140 mg/dl
➢ A1c of 6.5%

If you are relatively healthy and have some means and are relatively motivated, you can choose the "conventional control target".

Conventional Control Target (American Diabetes Association - ADA target):

➢ Fasting and before meals: 70-140 mg/dl
➢ 2 hours after meals <180 mg/dl
➢ A1c < 7.0%

If your personal and social resources are limited and are prone to having low sugar, your goal can be to achieve the reasonable control target.

Reasonable Control Target

➢ Fasting and before meals: 70-160 mg/dl, occasionally reaching 180 mg/dl
➢ 2 hours after meals <200 mg/dl
➢ A1c < 8.0%

If you have very limited means, are prone to having low sugar, and you are either older or have multiple debilitating diseases, then your goal is to prevent very low sugar and very high sugar. The target in this case is to avoid extremes or as I phrased it "No Extreme Target.".

No Extreme Target:

➢ Fasting and before meals: 70-200, very rarely to 300
➢ 2 hours after meals <300 mg/dl
➢ No A1c target

If you are pregnant, lots of organizations recommended a pregnant target. This is unrealistic for some patients. I always have a realistic achievable target for my patients. It is important to recognize that the chance of delivering a healthy baby goes up significantly if the mother's diabetes is well controlled.

Pregnant Target:

> ➢ Fasting, premeal, bedtime, and overnight glucose: 60-99 mg/dl
> ➢ After meal 100-120 mg/dl
> ➢ A1C ≤6%

Can I have a personalized day to day dose adjustment guideline?

If you are using basal insulin only, I presume you have type 2 diabetes. If you have type 1 diabetes, you should not use a basal insulin only regimen. Here we are talking about Basaglar, Lantus, Levemir, Toujeo, Tresiba used as a basal insulin in type 2 diabetes.

1. Again, you need to check your sugar two times a day, morning and bedtime.
2. You need to try your best to keep your activity and diet stable.
3. For most patients, after the stable dose has been reached, the dose does not need to be changed day to day.
4. There are even some doctors that believe your basal should be a set number.
5. However, since life is nothing but constant change, you might eat different foods, do different activities, or take different medications, or be in a different mood, or be in pain, etc. So your sugar will fluctuate. We want your sugar to fluctuate within a certain level only.

This can be your personalized day to day basal insulin dose adjustment recommendation. You can ask your doctor to fill it out for you.

Patient Name:

Insulin:

Date:

1. My usual daily stabilized full dose: given at:
    (morning, night)
2. My morning sugar target:
3. My bedtime sugar target:
4. Give   units if morning sugar: bedtime sugar:
5. Give   units, if morning sugar: bedtime sugar:
6. Give   units, if morning sugar: bedtime sugar:
7. Hold if morning sugar: bedtime sugar:

If your daily dose has to be changed day to day, you need to discuss your lifestyle, eating habits with your doctor. You might need to change your regimen.

Chapter 2. Glargine: Lantus/Basaglar

What is Lantus? What is Basaglar?

Both Lantus and Basaglar are human insulin analog glargine. They are engineered and commercially produced in bacteria. They are both long-acting insulin and used as basal insulin. They last 16-24 hours.

Basaglar is called a biosimilar product of Lantus. They are supposed to work the same way. In my experience, they seem to work comparably.

I have type 2 diabetes. My doctor started me on Lantus (or biosimilar Basaglar). Should I give it in the morning or night, before a meal or after a meal?

You can either give it in the morning or at night. If you always have higher sugars in the morning, I would recommend you give it at night; if you are prone to having low sugar at night, I would recommend you give it in the morning. Otherwise, you may take it in the morning or night.

Often, I recommend that patients give it two times a day. The benefit of doing this is:

- You have two chances to adjust your dose. The chance for low or high sugar can be reduced.
- Since Lantus or Basaglar does not really last 24 hours, if you give it two times a day, the level will be more stable. I and many endocrinologists tend to do this when the total Lantus or Basaglar dose is more than 50 units per day or sometimes the dose is very low.

- You can give it before or after the meal. Again, I recommend you stick to your schedule.

I have type 2 diabetes. My doctor wanted to start me on Lantus (or biosimilar Basaglar). What is the appropriate starting dose?

This actually depends on your sugar target, your sugar level, your weight, your kidney function and so on. However for new insulin users, for elderly or thin patients, I usually start with 15 units at night or in the morning. For younger patients 5-6 units two times a day is a reasonable approach. For more obese patients, I would start with 20-30 units.

I have type 2 diabetes, my doctor wanted to start me on Lantus (or biosimilar Basaglar), what is your recommendation for titrating the dose?

It is important to start on the right dose, but more important to titrate your dose based on your response. I want my patients to check sugar at least two times a day (morning and night), and stay on the same dose for 1 week, I usually start at a low dose, so the chance of having too low sugar is very rare. I usually do not recommend having very tight control in the beginning to avoid hypoglycemia. I think it is important for the patient to become familiar with the regimen first and as this occurs, the insulin dose can be increased as needed. If hypoglycemia occurs, I recommend you cut down your dose by half and stay on it for a week, and then begin to increase the dose gradually if needed.

Again, I ask patients to check sugar two times a day. If after a week, morning sugar is still above 130 mg/dl for two consecutive days then add 2 more units. I also give them a maximal dose such as 40 units or 60 units based on their body sizes and other factors including renal function and propensity toward having low sugar.

I have type 2 diabetes, and my doctor started me on Lantus or Basaglar once a day. How often should I check my sugar?

You have to check your sugar at least 2 times a day, morning and night. However, for many reasons, patients have excuses not to check or cut down the times to check. If you are one of these people, you can check once a day just before you give insulin. I frequently ask patients to check blood sugar fasting and bedtime alternating with lunch and supper so that I have a better idea of what their daily blood sugars are doing.

Do you recommend vial or pen?

If possible, I would recommend pen. The pen is so much easier to use, especially if you have vision issues or have tremors.

Basaglar only comes in a pen.

If I am using the pen, can I leave the needle on for the next injection?

It is not recommended to leave the needle on for the next injection. It might increase the risk for inaccuracy or infection. The needles are designed for one time use only. If use for second time. It is not as sharp as it should be. It cause more injury.

If I use the pen, should I leave the pen in the refrigerator or room temperature?

After you start using a new pen, you should leave it outside in a cool place that's not exposed to sun. You should not put it back in the refrigerator.

After I start to use the pen, how long can I use it?

After you start to use the pen, you need to discard it after 28 days even if you still have insulin left in the pen.

If I use the vial, can I put the vial back in the refrigerator after using it?

You can, but you do not need to. You can just leave them at cool place at room temperature. If you put it back in the refrigerator, you need to warm it up every use.

If I start to use the vial, how long can I use it?

Same as for pens. After you open the vial, you can use it for a maximum of 28 days. So every time you open a new vial, mark the date on it.

How long can I store unopened pens and vials?

You need to store them at 36-46 F in the refrigerator. They can never be frozen. If they've been frozen, you need to discard them. They can be stored until the expiration date.

How can I transport insulin?

You can transport Lantus or Basaglar as any other insulin, cool but not frozen. This is acceptable. Based on availability and how long the journey, you can use different ways to keep your insulin cool. You can use bags, wallets, fridges with freezer packs, ice, or some fancy designed bags, and boxes.

I am using Lantus or Basaglar, but my morning sugar is still way too high. What can I do?

There are many reasons for your elevated sugar. The most common reasons for your high morning sugar are as follows:

- You ate too much at dinner or you ate too late.
- You ate something "wrong" at dinner like pizza.

- If you gave Lantus or Basaglar in the morning, you can consider giving the Lantus or Basaglar at night. For the first dose of transition, you need to cut down your dose at least 50%, then afterwards, you can start to adjust your dose based on my previous recommendations.

   Example: you took 30 units in the morning on Monday. Tuesday morning before breakfast, your blood sugar is 220. You came to see me. We decided to move your Lantus time to night. First night (Tuesday night), you give 15 units. Wednesday morning, do not give any Lantus. Wednesday night, you give 30 units. After a few days, then you can begin to increase your Lantus dose based on morning and night sugar every 2 days. I usually recommend to increase Lantus dose by 2 units if morning sugar >130 for 2 days. The maximum dose is 60 units. If your dose is >60 units and sugar is still high. Usually we have to add other regimen if possible.

- You can also try to split the dose into two doses, half in the morning and half at night. Then you can adjust your night dose based on your morning sugar. If for two consecutive days, your morning sugar is still above 130 mg/dl, then you can increase 2 units every other day. If your dose is already above 60 units, you need to add other remedies like premeal insulin.

I am on Lantus/Basaglar, and my morning sugar is too low. What should I do?

Most likely you took too much insulin. Again, if you are on basal insulin. I would recommend you check your sugar at least twice a day, morning and night.

Sugar is always fluctuating, and low sugar can be life threatening, therefore, before you start insulin you need to have your sugar target and plan.

As we discussed elsewhere, sugar is not only determined by what you eat, how much you eat, and how you eat, but also determined by other medications, your emotional status, pain, sleep, and your level of activity, etc.. Sugar can fluctuate day to day. You should always have a plan.

For details, please see the question "how do I adjust my basal insulin?"

I want to eat a big meal, can I give more Lantus or Basaglar?

Lantus or Basaglar are long-acting insulins. It is really not ideal to use the long-acting insulin to cover the meal. Overeating is not a good idea anyway.

I was hospitalized recently; the hospital used Levemir on me, but I have Lantus (or Basaglar) at home. What should I do?

If you were given a dose once a day in the hospital, you should be given the same dose at the same time using Lantus (or Basaglar). You can try one unit to one unit conversion from Levemir to Lantus or Basaglar.

If you were given Levemir two times a day in the hospital (which is more common than once daily) , one option is to use Lantus or Basaglar at the same dose and same time and same requency as Levemir (in this case twice a day such as breakfast and bedtime); another options is that if you want to get back to your previous one shot of Lantus or Basaglar, I recommend you use half of your first dose of your previous Lantus or Basaglar dosage to prevent the possibility of low sugar. The second day you can use the full dose (combine the two doses of Levemir).

For example: you are hospitalized and started on Levemir 15 units two times a day, but you have Lantus or Basaglar at home. One option is to use Lantus or Basaglar 15 units two times a day. If you rather get back to once a day. Your first night home, you need to use 15 units. The second morning, do not take it. Second night, you start to take 30 units. After a few days, then you can began to adjust your dose if your sugar is still high.

Most important is that you should ask your physician for specific advice and follow up with your physician.

My insurance changed my coverage from Levemir to Lantus or Basaglar. What can I do?

See the above answer.

I was using Humulin N (Novolin N) two times a day. Now my doctor has changed it to Lantus or Basaglar. What should I do?

I am glad you are changing to Lantus or Basaglar. Lantus or Basaglar can give you a much flatter insulin level. It is also so much easier to give. There is much less variation.

- First calculate the total dose of N you are taking.
- First day of conversion, I recommend you to take a half dose of total dose of N using Lantus or Basaglar.
- Then, after two to three days, depending on your regimen, once or twice a day, you can adjust your insulin dose based on the morning sugar. If for consecutive two days, your sugar is greater than 130, you can increase your Lantus or Basaglar by 2 units.
- You can have different targets based on your sugar stability and overall risks.

If your dose is greater than 60 units, I recommend you discuss other strategies with your doctor that keep your sugar under better control.

I am on premixed insulin (like Novolin 70/30, Humulin 70/30, Humalog 75/25, Humalog 50/50, Novolog 70/30), and now my doctor wants to switch me to Lantus or Basaglar. What should I do?

You might need more insulin than just basal insulin like Lantus or Basaglar, you might need to have some premeal insulin, like Humalog, Novolog, Apidra or Fiasp. If you have type 2 diabetes and want to try just basal insulin, I would recommend you do the same as if changing from N to Lantus or Basaglar. Please see above answer. If your physician gives specific instructions for you, you certainly should follow.

My insurance wants me to change Lantus to Basaglar. What should I do?

Presumably, you can just do one unit to one unit conversion. You can do the same if your insurance wants to change Basaglar to Lantus. These two insulins are equivalent.

My insurance wants me to change Toujeo to Lantus or Basaglar. What can I do?

Toujeo is also an insulin analog-glargine but 3 times as concentrated. It works slightly differently. I recommend starting with ¾ of the Toujeo dose using Lantus or Basaglar, and then titrate the dose based on fasting sugar. Again, increase the

Lantus or Basaglar dose by 2 units every two days if morning sugar is greater than 130 mg/dl, and reduce by 2 units if morning sugar is less than 100 mg/dl for 2 consecutive days. The final dose is usually an 80% dose of Toujeo.

The target can be different for different patients. You need to discuss this with your doctor.

My insurance wants me to change from Tresiba to Lantus or Basaglar. What should I do?

Tresiba is another basal insulin and lasts much longer. It lasts more than 24 hours and up to 42 hours. I recommend you do the same as with converting Toujeo to Lantus or Basaglar. For the first day, you should start with half or ¾ of the dose of Tresiba using Lantus or Basaglar, and then adjust the dose based on your morning sugar. You can increase the Lantus or Basaglar dose by 2 units if your morning sugar is greater than 130 for 2 consecutive days, and reduce by two units if your morning sugar is less than 100 for 2 consecutive days. Your final dose of Lantus or Basaglar is usually 80% of a Tresiba dose.

Your target can be different based on your sugar stability and overall risks. If you and your doctor decide on tighter control, you can set your target at 100. For example, you can increase your insulin dose 2 units every two days if your sugar is over 100, and reduce 2 units every two days if your sugar is less than 80.

What else is in Lantus?

The active ingredient is glargine.

Inactive ingredients for the 10 mL vial are 30 mcg zinc, 2.7 mg m-cresol, 20 mg glycerol 85%, 20 mcg polysorbate 20, and water for injection.

What is m-cresol? Is it toxic?

It is a derivative of phenol and is an isomer of p-cresol and o-crestol. Together with many other compounds, m-cresol is traditionally extracted from coal tar.

The synonyms are: 1-Hydroxy-3-methylbenzene; 3-Cresol; 3-Hydroxytoluene; 3-Methylphenol; m-Cresole; m-Cresylic acid; m-Hydroxytoluene; m-Kresol; m-Methylphenol; m-Oxytoluene; m-Toluol; phenol, 3-methyl-; Metacresol.

It is used as a preservative. It is certainly toxic. Some patients' adverse reactions to Lantus might be related to an reaction to m-cresol. Skin inflammation is characterized by itching, scaling, reddening, or occasionally blistering.

It might be carcinogenic, which means it might cause cancer. It might also cause damage to your central nervous system (brain and spinal cord), liver, kidney, and so on.

What is polysorbate-20? Is it toxic?

Polysorbate-20 is Tween 20 to many people like me. I used to do lots of laboratory research. We use it to lyse cells, make washing solution, block binding sites, solubilize proteins, and so on. It is 20 repeat units of polyethylene glycol. It is relatively safe. Certainly you need to ingest as little as possible.

Should I stop Lantus since it contains toxic substances?

You should not. First, you need it. The benefit of using it far outweighs not using it. You need to discuss with your doctor before stopping; Second, I recommend you use the lowest dose possible. That is why I strongly urge you to eat right and exercise. (For more information about how to treat diabetes, please read my other book about diabetes management <<Diabetes Questions and Answers More Than 400 Diabetes Frequently Asked Questions>>)

If I am allergic to Lantus or Basaglar, what options do I have?

Allergies (hypersensitivity) can occur with any medication including insulin Lantus or Basaglar. Luckily, we have many choices these days. You can try Levemir, or Tresiba. Toujeo is not a good choice since Toujeo is also glargine which is the same active ingredient in Lantus or Basaglar.

If none of above work, you can use an insulin pump or V-go to deliver both basal and bolus insulin using fast-acting insulin like Humalog, Novolog, Apidra or Fiasp.

I have never had to desensitize any patient.

Chapter 3. Glargine: Toujeo

What is Toujeo?

Toujeo is like Lantus which is insulin glargine, but 3 times as concentrated. It is only available as a pen (Toujeo SoloStar insulin glargine injection. U-300). It reduces your injection volume, but since it is only provided as a pen, you do not need to worry about that. You use it as you would any other insulin: just based on units. You do not need to consider volume adjustment. Do not try to do any calculations.

We use Toujeo as basal long-acting insulin. It lasts over 24 hours.

Is Toujeo better than Lantus or Basaglar?

Every kind of insulin has its place in treating diabetes. At some certain points, Toujeo may be better for some patients; and at other certain points, Toujeo may not be advantageous.

I have type 2 diabetes and my doctor started me on Toujeo. Should I give it in the morning or night?

You can either give it in the morning or at night, As a matter of fact, you might use it any time of the day, before meals or after. I do recommend you give at the same time of every day.

If you always have high sugars in the morning, I recommend to give at night; if you are prone to having low sugar during the night, I recommend to give it in the morning. Otherwise, you can take it in the morning or night.

The Toujeo pen can give a maximum dose of 80 units. If your dose is more than 80 units, then you have to give two shots. If this is the case, I recommend you give it twice a day, one in the morning and one at night.

You will have two chances to adjust your dose. The chance for low or too high sugar can be reduced.

I usually also recommend you to start premeal insulin or other non-insulin injections like GLP-1 agonist if you need more than 80 units. I consider premeal insulin if your dose is more than 60 units.

I have type 2 diabetes, and my doctor wanted to start me on Toujeo. What is the appropriate starting dose?

This actually depends on your sugar target, your sugar level, your weight, your kidney function and so on. However, for new insulin users, for elderly or thin patients, I usually start with 15-20 units at night or morning. For younger or more obese patients, I would start with 30 units. Since Toujeo is 3 times as concentrated as Lantus, I would not recommend Toujeo to patients whose insulin dose is below 15 units because if the dose is lower, the dose error is increased. If your doctor says you might not need 15 units, you should be started on other insulins like Lantus, Levemir, or Basaglar.

I have type 2 diabetes and my doctor wanted to start me on Toujeo, what is your recommendation for titrating the dose?

It is important to start on the right dose, but more important to titrate your dose based on your responses. I want my patient to check sugar at least two times a day morning and night, and stay on the same dose for one week if their sugar is not too low. I usually do not recommend having very tight control in the beginning to avoid hypoglycemia and to let the patient become familiar with the regimen.

Again, I ask patient to check sugar twice a day. If after a week, morning sugar is still above 130 mg/dl for 3 consecutive days, then add 3 more units. I also give them a maximal dose for example 60 units or 80 units, based on their body size and other conditions.

As we discussed, your target can be 100, 130 or 160 depending on your sugar stability and overall risk. You and your doctor need to make the decision together.

I usually do not recommend basal insulin only treatment over 60 units. If your basal insulin needs are over 60 units and your sugar is still not under target control, I would recommend adding on treatments like premeal bolus shots.

I was started on Toujeo, and now I am pregnant. What should I do?

Toujeo has not been licensed to be used in pregnant woman. However, you do not need to panic or stop Toujeo right away. I recommend you call your doctor and let him or her know, so your regimen can be changed. Before you see your doctor, do not stop your treatment.

Again, Toujeo is not licensed to be used on pregnant women which does not mean there is danger to the fetus immediately. Toujeo has not been studied in pregnant women.

Do you recommend vial or pen?

Toujeo only comes as a pen.

If I am using the pen, can I leave the needle on for the next injection?

It is not recommended to leave the needle on for the next injection. It might increase the risk for inaccuracy and infection. It can cause insulin leaking. The reused needle might cause more injection injury and cause scar.

Should I leave the Toujeo pen in the refrigerator or outside at room temperature?

After starting a new pen, you should leave it outside of the refrigerator in a cool place that's not exposed to sun. You should not put it back in the refrigerator.

After I start a new pen, how long can I use it?

After you started a new pen, you need to discard it after 42 days even if you still have insulin left in the pen. Every pen has 450 units of insulin (1.5 cc).

How long can I store the unopened pens of Toujeo?

You need to store them at 36-46 F in the refrigerator. They should never be frozen. If frozen, you need to discard them. They can be stored until the expiration date.

How can I transport insulin Toujeo?

Transport Toujeo as you would do any other insulin. They need to be kept cool but not frozen. Based on availability and how long the journey, you can try different ways to keep your insulin cool. You can use bags, wallets, fridges with freezer packs, ice, or some specially designed bags or boxes.

I am using Toujeo but my morning sugar is still way too high. What can I do?

There are many reasons for your elevated sugar. The most common reason for your high morning sugar is as follows:

- Ate too much at dinner and/or ate too late.
- Ate something "wrong" at dinner like pizza.
- If you give Toujeo in the morning, you can consider giving it at night. For the first day of transition, you need to reduce your dose by at least 50%, then afterwards, you can start to adjust your dose based on my recommendation as follows:

  I recommend you adjust your dose after using Toujeo for a week, then every 3 days, based on your morning sugars and night sugar, titrate your dose. If both your morning and night sugars are greater than 130 for 3 consecutive days, you can increase your insulin by 2-3 units. I recommend a maximum dose of 60-80 units. The maximum one injection pen can deliver is 80 units.

- If your dose is at the maximum dose already, you need to add another remedy like premeal insulin.

I want to eat a big meal. Can I give more Toujeo?

Toujeo is a long acting insulin. It is not really ideal to use long acting insulin to cover a meal. Overeating is not a good idea at any time.

I was hospitalized recently and the hospital used Lantus/or Basaglar or Levemir on me, but I use Toujeo at home. What should I do?

If you were given those once a day in the hospital, you should give the same dose at the same time using Toujeo. Be aware, for the first 3 days, your sugar might be slightly higher. Again I recommend titrating your Toujeo after a week.

If you were given Levemir/Lantus/Basaglar twice a day in the hospital, one option is to use the same dose of Toujeo at the same time as Lantus/Basaglar/Levemir. Another option is to get back to your previous one shot of Toujeo, if you want. For the first dose, I recommend using half of your previous hospital Lantus/Basaglar/Levemir dose to prevent the possibility of low sugar. For the second dose, you can use the full dose. Then after a week on Toujeo, you can start to titrate your dose if your sugar is not low. If your sugar is too low (especially if your morning sugar<70 mg/dl), you need to reduce your dose by half and if your sugar is still less than 70 mg/dl, you need to reduce your dose by half again until your sugar is above 100 mg/dl. Then after a week begin to titrate.

My insurance changed my coverage from Lantus, Basaglar, or Levemir to Toujeo. What can I do?

See the above answer.

I was using Humulin N (Novolin N) 2 times a day. Now my doctor changed it to Toujeo. What should I do?

I am glad that you are changing to Toujeo. Toujeo can give you a much flatter insulin level. It is also much easier to give. There is also much less variation.

- First calculate the total dose of N you are taking.
- First day of transition, I recommend taking a half dose of N insulin using Toujeo.
- Then, after a few days or a week, depending of your regimen, you can adjust your insulin dose based on your morning and bedtime sugar. If your sugar >130 mg/dl for 3 consecutive days, you can increase your Toujeo by 3 units every 3 days.

If your dose is greater than 60-80 units, I recommend discussing with your doctor other things you need to do to get your sugar under better control.

I am on a premix insulin like Novolin 70/30, Humulin 70/30, Humalog 75/25, Novolog 70/30, and now my doctor wants to switch me to Toujeo. What should I do?

If you were on premix before, you might need more insulin than just basal insulin like Toujeo. You might need to have some premeal insulin, like Humalog, Novolog, Fiasp, or Apidra.

If you have type 2 diabetes and just want to try basal insulin only, I would recommend doing the same as converting N to Toujeo. If you have type 1 diabetes, you cannot be on basal insulin only regimen.

- First calculate the total dose of premix you are taking.
- For the first day of transition, I recommend you take a half dose of premix insulin using Toujeo.
- Then, after a few days or a week, depending on your regimen, you can adjust your insulin dose based on your morning and bedtime sugar. If your sugar >130 mg/dl for 3 consecutive days, you can increase your Toujeo by 3 units every 3 days if your sugar is still high.

If your sugar is too low, you certainly need to reduce your dose. The chance to be too low is relative small since we started half of your previous insulin dose. However, if you have too low sugar (<70), I recommend you reduce your insulin dose by another 50% and then titrate based on my scheme.

If your dose is greater than 60-80 units, I recommend discussing with your doctor other things you need to do to get your sugar under better control.

My insurance wants me to change from Tresiba to Toujeo. What should I do?

Tresiba is another basal insulin and lasts much longer. It lasts from 24 hours up to 42 hours. For your first week, you should start with 80% of the dose of Tresiba using Toujeo, and then adjust the dose based on the morning and bedtime sugar. After one week, you can increase the Toujeo dose by 2 units if your morning and bedtime sugar is greater than 130 for three consecutive days, and reduce by 2 units if your morning sugar is less than 80 for two consecutive days. If you have a sugar lower than 60, I recommend to reduce by 50%. Your final dose of Toujeo is usually the same dose of Tresiba.

What else is in Toujeo?

Inactive ingredients for the 1.5 mL Toujeo pen per ml are 90 mcg zinc, 2.7 mg m-cresol, 20 mg glycerol 85%, and water for injection.

What is m-cresol? Is it toxic?

It is a derivative of phenol and is an isomer of p-cresol and o-cresol. Together with many other compounds, m-cresol is traditionally extracted from coal tar.

The synonyms are: 1-Hydroxy-3-methylbenzene; 3-Cresol; 3-Hydroxytoluene; 3-Methylphenol; m-Cresole; m-Cresylic acid; m-Hydroxytoluene; m-Kresol; m-Methylphenol; m-Oxytoluene; m-Toluol; phenol, 3-methyl-; Metacresol.

It is used as a preservative. It is certainly toxic. Some patients having adverse reactions to Toujeo might be related to m-cresol. Skin inflammation is characterized by itching, scaling, reddening, or, occasionally blistering.

It might be carcinogenic, which means it might cause cancer. It might also cause damage to your central nervous system (brain and spinal cord), liver, kidneys and so on.

Should I stop Toujeo since it contains toxic substances?

You should not. First, you need it. The benefit of using it far outweighs not using it. You need to discuss with your doctor before stopping it. Second, I *do* recommend using the lowest dose possible. That is why I strongly urge you to eat right and exercise. (For more information about how to treat diabetes, please read my other book about diabetes management <<Diabetes Questions and Answers More Than 400 Diabetes Frequently Asked Questions>>).

If I am allergic to Toujeo, what options do I have?

Allergy (oversensitivity) can occur with any medication. You might have minor reactions like itching, rash and so on. Major reactions can cause shortness of breath or anaphylaxis (shock) and can be life threatening.

Under close supervision, you might want to try different insulins like Levemir, or Tresiba. Lantus or Basaglar are not good choices, since they contain the same active ingredient glargine as Toujeo.

If you are still having trouble, I recommend using an insulin pump or V-go to deliver fast-acting insulin like Humalog, Novolog, Apidra or Fiasp for your basal and bolus insulin needs.

Chapter 4 : Levemir

What is Levemir?

Levemir is human insulin analog. It was engineered and commercially produced in specialized, modified yeast. It is a long-acting insulin and used as basal insulin. It lasts 16-24 hours.

I have type 2 diabetes and my doctor started me on Levemir. Should I give it in the morning or night?

You can give it either in the morning or at night. You can give it before or after a meal. If you always have higher sugars in the morning, I would recommend giving it at night; if you are prone to having low sugar during the night, I would recommend giving it in the morning. Otherwise, you can take it in the morning or night.

Frequently, I recommend patients give Levemir twice a day. The benefit of doing this is:

- You have two chances to adjust your dose. The chance for either low sugar or too high can be reduced.
- Since Levemir doesn't really last 24 hours, if you do it twice a day, the level will be more stable.

I have type 2 diabetes and my doctor wanted to start me on Levemir. What is the appropriate starting dose?

This actually depends on your sugar target, your sugar level, your weight, your kidney function, your liver function, and so on. However, for new insulin users, for elderly or thin patients, I usually start with 10 units at night or morning. For younger and more obese patients, I would start with 20-30 units. Again, I might recommend splitting the dose (morning and night).

I have type 2 diabetes and my doctor wants to start me on Levemir. What is your recommendation for titrating the dose?

It is important to start on the right dose, but more important to titrate your dose based on your responses. I want my patients to check sugar at least twice a day, morning and night, and stay on the same dose for one week. I usually do not recommend having very tight control in the beginning to avoid hypoglycemia and let my patients become familiar with the regimen.

Again, I ask patients to check sugar twice a day. If after a week, both morning and night sugars are still above 130 mg/dl for two consecutive days, add 2 more units. I also give them a maximum dose like 40 units or 60 units based on their body sizes and other medical conditions like heart disease or liver kidney diseases.

Please review it with your treating physician. I have a personalized recommendation in Chapter 1.

Do you recommend vial or pen?

If possible, I would recommend pen. The pen is much easier to use especially if you have vision issues or have tremors.

After I start using a new pen, how long can I use it?

You need to discard it 28 days from the start day even if you still have insulin left in the pen.

If I use the vial, can I put the vial back in the refrigerator after each use?

You can, but you do not need to. You can just leave it in a cool place at room temperature. If you put it back in the refrigerator, you need to warm it up to room temperature before using each time.

If I start to use the vial, how long can I use it?

Same as for a pen. After you open the vial, the maximum days you can use it is 28 days. So when you open a new vial, mark the date on it.

How long can I store the unopened pens and vials?

You need to store them at 36-46 F in the refrigerator. They should never be frozen. If frozen, you need to discard them. They can be stored until their expiration date.

How can I transport Levemir?

You can transport Levemir like any other insulin. As long as you keep them cool but not frozen, they will be acceptable. Based on availability and how long the journey, you can use different ways to keep your insulin cool. You can use bags, wallets, fridges with freezer packs, ice, or some fancy designer bags, and boxes.

I am using Levemir and my morning sugar is still way too high. What should I do?

There are many reasons for your elevated sugar. The most common reasons for your high morning sugar are as follows:

- Ate too much at dinner and/or ate too late.
- Ate something "wrong" at dinner like pizza.
- If you give Levemir in the morning, you can consider giving it at night. For the first day of transition, you need to cut down your dose by at least 50%, then afterwards, you can start to adjust your dose based on my previous recommendations.
- You can also try to split the dose into two doses, half in the morning and half at night. Then you can adjust your night dose based on your morning sugar. You can increase your night time dose by 2 units every other day if your morning sugar has not reached your target.

I want to eat a big meal, can I give more Levemir?

Levemir is a long-acting insulin. It is really not ideal to use the long-acting insulin to cover the meal. Overeating is not a good idea anyway.

If you are planning on feasting for extended hours, you may try giving 30-50% more of your dose in the morning 1-2 hours before your feast begins. Again, I am not promoting overeating. You always have to control your diet even on holidays.

I was hospitalized recently and the hospital used Lantus or Basaglar on me, but I use Levemir at home. What should I do?

If you were given Lantus/Basaglar once a day in the hospital, you can try to giving the same dose at same time using Levemir. However, usually I like to prescribe Levemir two times a day. You can start your first half dose 24 hours after your last dose of Lantus or Basaglar. For the first day your sugar might be slightly high, but it is okay. It might take three to four days to stabilize to the new dose of Levemir.

If you were given Lantus/Basaglar two times a day in the hospital, then it is perfect. I like to use Levemir two times a day any way. You can just do one unit to one unit switch.

If your insurance covers Lantus or Basaglar, you might switch to the same insulin as your local hospital is using. Then, you do not have to worry about it in case you are hospitalized again.

My insurance changed my coverage from Lantus or Basaglar to Levemir. What can I do?

See the above answer.

I was using Humulin N (Novolin N) twice a day. Now my doctor has changed it to Levemir. What should I do?

I am glad that you are changing to Levemir. Levemir can give you a much more flatter insulin level. It is also so much easier to give. The variation is also much less.

- First calculate the total dose of N you are taking.
- For the first day of transition, I recommend you to take 50% of the dose.
- Then, after two or three days, if your sugar is too high, you can adjust your insulin dose based on the morning and night sugar. Different patients have different targets. If your morning and night sugar target are 130, then if for two consecutive days your sugar is greater than 130, you can increase your Levemir by 2 units.

If your dose is greater than 60 units, I recommend discussing with your doctor other things you need to do to get your sugar under better control.

I am on premix insulin like Novolin 70/30, Humulin 70/30, Humalog 75/25, Humalog 50/50, or Novolog 70/30, and now my doctor wants to switch me to Levemir. What should I do?

If you were on premix before, you might need more insulin than just basal insulin like Levemir. You might need to have some premeal insulin, like Humalog, Novolog, Fiasp, or Apidra. If you have type 1 diabetes, then you have to take premeal short-acting insulin.

If you have type 2 diabetes and just want to try basal insulin, I would recommend the following strategy:

- First calculate the total dose of premix insulin you are taking.
- For the first day of transition, I recommend you to take 50% of the dose using Levemir.
- Then, after two or three days, if your sugar is too high, you can adjust your insulin dose based on the morning and night sugar. Different patients have different targets. If your morning and night sugar target are 130, then if for two consecutive days your sugar is greater than 130, you can increase your Levemir by 2 units.
- If you sugar drops below 70, you need to reduce the dose by 50% and then begin to titrate again.
- If your dose is greater than 60 units, I recommend discussing with your doctor other things you need to do to get your sugar under better control.

My insurance wants me to change from Toujeo to Levemir. What can I do?

Toujeo is also an insulin analog-glargine but three times as concentrated. It works slightly different. I recommend starting at 50-80% of the Toujeo dose using Levemir, then titrating the dose based on fasting sugar. Again, increase the Levemir dose by 2 units every two days, if your morning sugars are greater than 130 (if 130 is your target), and reduce by 2 units if your morning sugars are less than 100 for two consecutive days. The final dose usually is 80% dose of the Toujeo dose. You might have different target. You need to discuss with your doctor.

My insurance wants me to change from Tresiba to Levemir. What should I do?

Tresiba is another basal insulin and lasts much longer. It lasts from 24 to 42 hours. I recommend you do the same as for transitioning from Toujeo to Levemir. For the first day, you should start with a 50% of previous dose of Tresiba using Levemir, and then adjust the dose based on the morning sugar. You can increase the Levemir dose by 2 units if your morning sugars are greater than 130 for two consecutive days, and reduce two units if your morning sugar less than 100 for two consecutive days. Your final dose of Levemir is usually 80% of the Tresiba dose. Again, you can choose a different target based on your own specific situation.

What else is in Levemir?

Each milliliter of Levemir contains 100 U (14.2 mg/mL) of insulin detemir. Each milliliter of Levemir 10 mL Vial contains inactive ingredients: 65.4 mcg zinc, 2.06 mg m-cresol, 30.0 mg mannitol, 1.80 mg phenol, 0.89 mg disodium phosphate dihydrate, 1.17 mg sodium chloride, and water for injection.

What is m-cresol? Is it toxic?

It is a derivative of phenol and is an isomer of p-cresol and o-cresol. Together with many other compounds, m-cresol is traditionally extracted from coal tar.

The synonyms are: 1-Hydroxy-3-methylbenzene; 3-Cresol; 3-Hydroxytoluene; 3-Methylphenol; m-Cresole; m-Cresylic acid; m-Hydroxytoluene; m-Kresol; m-Methylphenol; m-Oxytoluene; m-Toluol; phenol, 3-methyl; Metacresol.

It is used as a preservative and certainly is toxic. Some patients' adverse reaction to Levemir might be because of a reaction to m-cresol. Skin inflammation is characterized by itching, scaling, reddening, or occasionally blistering.

It might be carcinogenic, meaning it might cause cancer. It might also cause damage to your central nervous system (brain and spinal cord), liver, kidneys and so on.

What is mannitol? Is it toxic?

Mannitol is a sugar alcohol. It is not toxic, especially at this level.

Should I stop Levemir since it contains toxic substance?

You should not. First, you need it. The benefit of using it far outweighs not using it. You need to discuss with your doctor before stopping it. Second, I recommend you use the lowest dose possible. That is why I strongly urge you to eat right and exercise. (for more information about treating diabetes, please read my other book about diabetes management <<Diabetes Questions and Answers More Than 400 Diabetes Frequently Asked Questions>>)

If I am allergic to Levemir, what options do I have?

You can try other options like Lantus, Basaglar, Tresiba, or use fast-acting insulins like Humalog, Novolog, Fiasp, Apidra, or regular insulin using an insulin pump or V-go to deliver your insulin.

If you have type 2 diabetes, you really need to read my other book <<Diabetes Questions and Answers More Than 400 Diabetes Frequently Asked Questions>>. You learn more about diabetes and strive to live better. You might not need any insulin at all.

If you are still allergic to these options, then you might have to become desensitized. Fortunately, this is rare.

Chapter 5 : Tresiba

What is Tresiba?

Tresiba is human insulin analog degludec. It was engineered and commercially produced in specialized yeast and then chemically modified to add a C16 fatty acid to insulin molecule. It is a long-acting insulin and used as basal insulin. Its effect can last at least 42 hours.

Should I give it in the morning or night?

You can either give it in the morning or at night. As a matter of fact, you can give at any time of the day, before a meal or after a meal.

I have type 2 diabetes, and my doctor wants to start me on Tresiba. What is the appropriate starting dose?

This actually depends on your sugar target, your sugar level, your weight, your kidney function, your liver function, and so on. However, for new insulin users, for elderly or thin patients, I usually start with 10-16 units at night or morning. For younger or more obese patients, I would start with 20-30 units.

If you are on insulin already, I recommend reducing 20% of your total dose, then start to adjust your dose after one week if your sugar is high. You need to cut down the dose if you have low sugar.

I have type 2 diabetes and my doctor wanted to start me on Tresiba. What is your recommendation for titrating the dose?

It is important to start on the right dose, but more important to titrate your dose based on your responses. I want my patients to check their sugar at least two times a day (morning and night), and stay on the same dose for one week. I usually do not recommend having very tight control in the beginning to avoid hypoglycemia and to let patients become familiar with the regimen.

Again, I ask patients to check their sugars two times a day. If after a week, both morning and night sugars are still above 130 mg/dl for three to four consecutive days, add 2 more units. I also give them a maximum dose like 40-80 units based on their body sizes.

Tresiba can take one week to reach a stable status. Therefore do not start to titrate the dose too early, and do not titrate the dose too often.

Please review it with your physician.

Do you recommend a vial or pen?

Tresiba only comes in a pen: Tresiba U-100, or U-200. The U-100 pen has 300 units; while the U-200 Pen has 600 units.

The U-100 of Tresiba comes in a five-pen box; while U-200 of Tresiba comes in a three-pen box. The maximum dose of U-100 in one injection is 80 units; while the maximum dose of U-200 in one injection is 160 units.

For some reason, I have both U-100 and U-200 pens. What should I pay attention to when I do the injection?

Remember that when you do the injection with a pen, you do not need to worry about U-100 or U-200. The only thing you need to pay attention to is the units. This rule applies to other insulins too, like Toujeo U-300 or Humulin R U-500 pen.

If I am using the pen, can I leave the needle on for the next injection?

It is not recommended to leave the needle on for the next injection. It might increase the risk for inaccuracy and infection or injection injury.

If I use the pen, should I leave the pen in the refrigerator or at room temperature?

After you start to use a pen, you should leave it outside in a cool place and not exposed to the sun. You should not put it back in the refrigerator.

After I start using a new pen, how long can I use it?

After you start using a new pen, you need to discard it after 56 days even if you still have insulin left in the pen. If you use up one pen before starting a new pen, you should not have to worry about this.

How long can I store the unopened pens?

You need to store them at 36-46 F in the refrigerator. They should never be frozen. If frozen, you need to discard them. They can be stored until their expiration date.

How long can I store the unopened pen at room temperature?

You should store unopened pens in a refrigerator. If you do not have access to a refrigerator, you can store an unopened pen at room temperature for 56 days.

How can I transport Tresiba insulin?

You can transport Tresiba like any other insulin. As long as you keep it cool but not frozen, it will be acceptable. Based on availability and how long the journey, you can use different ways to keep your insulin cool. You can use bags, wallets, fridges with freezer packs, ice, or some fancy designed bags, and boxes.

However, if you are just on a short trip, and the temperature is below 86 F (30 C). You can transport either an opened or unopened pen without a special bag or box, or cooler. You can use either opened or unopened pens up to 56 days.

I am using Tresiba and my morning sugar is still way too high.

There are many reasons for your elevated sugar. The most common reasons for your high morning sugar are as follows:

- Ate too much at dinner and/or ate too late.
- Ate something" wrong" at dinner like pizza.
- Here's what you can do:
    a. Take a walk after your dinner.
    b. A week after you start your Tresiba insulin, you can start to titrate your dose. You can increase your dose by 2 units every three or four days if your morning sugar is still above your target, and your bedtime sugar is above 130 mg/dl.
- Your doctor might have a different target for you. You need to discuss with your doctor in more detail.

I want to eat a big meal. Can I give more Tresiba?

Tresiba is a long-acting insulin. It is really not ideal to use the long-acting insulin to cover the meal. Overeating is not a good idea anyway.

Although after a single injection, it begins to work after one hour. Tresiba takes three to four days and up to seven days to reach a steady status.

I was hospitalized recently, and the hospital used Lantus, Basaglar or Levemir on me. I have Tresiba at home. What should I do?

If you were given Lantus/Basaglar or Levemir once a day in the hospital, you can try to give the same dose at the same time using Tresiba. However, if you were given basal insulin two times a day in the hospital, you can combine the dose and give one dose of Tresiba. I recommend to give 24 hour after last dose of Lantus, Basaglar, or Levemir in the hospital.

My insurance changed my coverage from Lantus, Basaglar, or Levemir to Tresiba. What can I do?

If you were given Lantus, Basaglar or Levemir once a day before, and the dose is less than 80 units daily, you can try to give the same dose at the same time using Tresiba. However, if you were given basal insulin two times a day before and total dose is more than 80 units, you can just start at the same dose at the same time for Tresiba. You can also combine the doses using the Tresiba U-200. However, I strongly recommend your doctor review your regimen. If your total dose is less than 80 units, and you would like to combine two doses into one dose, you need to give Tresiba 24 hours after your last dose of basal insulin. The first dose after switching, your sugar might be elevated, but it is fine. It takes three to four days or even up to seven days for Tresiba to reach a steady status.

I was using Humulin N (Novolin N) twice a day and now my doctor has changed it to Tresiba. What should I do?

I am glad you are changing to Tresiba. Tresiba can give you a much flatter insulin level.

- First calculate the total dose of N you are taking.
- For the first day of transition, I recommend you take 50% of the combined dose using Tresiba.
- After one week, you can adjust your insulin dose based on the morning and night sugar. Different patients have different targets; if your morning and night sugar targets are 130; if your sugar is greater than 130 for three to four days consecutively, you can increase your Tresiba by 2 units.
- If your dose is greater than 80 units, I recommend you discuss with your doctor to see if there are any other medications you need to meet your sugar target.

I am on premix insulin like Novolin 70/30, Humulin 70/30, Humalog 75/25, or Novolog 70/30, and now my doctor wants to switch me to Tresiba. What should I do?

If you were on premix before, you might need more insulin than just basal insulin like Tresiba. You might need to have some premeal insulin, like Humalog, Novolog, Apidra, Fiasp or regular insulin. If you have type 1 diabetes, then you definitely need premeal insulin (short-acting, fast-acting).

If you have type 2 diabetes and just want to try basal insulin, I would recommend doing the same as converting N to Tresiba as above.

- First calculate the total dose of premix you are taking.
- For the first day of transition, I recommend you take 50% of the combined dose.

- After one week, you can adjust your insulin dose based on the morning and night sugar. Different patients have different targets; if your morning and night sugar target is 130, then if your sugar is greater than 130 for three to four days consecutively, you can increase your Tresiba by 2 units.
- If your sugar is less than 100, then you can reduce by 2-3 units every day. If your sugar less than 70, I recommend to reduce by 50% for next dose and titrate again.

My insurance wants me to change from Toujeo to Tresiba. What can I do?

Toujeo is another insulin analog-glargine but three times as concentrated as Lantus or Basaglar. It works slightly differently. I recommend reducing the insulin dose by 20% at the beginning of the switch. If your morning sugar is greater than 130 (if 130 is your target) after one week, increase the Tresiba dose by 2 units every three to four days; reduce by 2 units if your morning sugar is less than 100 for three consecutive days. Usually the maximum dose is 60-80 units. You can set a different target and different maximum dose.

My insurance wants me to change from Levemir to Tresiba. What should I do?

Levemir is a long-acting insulin that is also used as basal insulin. It lasts much less time. I usually like to use it twice a day. Tresiba is another basal insulin and lasts much longer. It lasts more than 24 hours and up to 42 hours.

First, calculate the total daily dose of Levemir. I recommend reducing your dose by 20% at the beginning of the transition. For the first day, you should start at 80% of the total dose of Levemir using Tresiba, and then after one week, you can start to adjust the dose based on the morning sugar. You can increase the Tresiba dose by 2 units if your morning sugar is greater than 130 for three consecutive days, and reduce by two units if your morning sugar is less than 100 for three consecutive days. If your morning sugar is less than 70, you need to cut the dose by half. Your final maximum dose of Tresiba should be less than 80 units.

Again, your target can be different based on your special circumstances. You need to discuss with your doctor in more detail. Please also read the section for "how to adjust the basal insulin" section.

If you need more than 80 units, you should be advised to start premeal insulin or in combination with other therapy.

What else is in Tresiba?

Each milliliter of Tresiba contains glycerol 19.6 mg, phenol 1.50 mg, metacresol 1.72 mg, zinc 32.7 mcg and water for injection.

What is metacresol (m-cresol)? Is it toxic?

It is a derivative of phenol and is an isomer of p-cresol and o-cresol. Together with many other compounds, m-cresol is traditionally extracted from coal tar.

The synonyms are: 1-Hydroxy-3-methylbenzene; 3-Cresol; 3-Hydroxytoluene; 3-Methylphenol; m-Cresole; m-Cresylic acid; m-Hydroxytoluene; m-Kresol; m-Methylphenol; m-Oxytoluene; m-Toluol; phenol, 3-methyl; Metacresol.

It is used as a preservative and certainly is toxic. Some patients' adverse reactions to Tresiba might be related to a reaction to m-cresol. Skin inflammation is characterized by itching, scaling, reddening, or, occasionally blistering.

It might be carcinogenic, meaning it might cause cancer. It might also cause damage to your central nervous system (brain and spinal cord), liver, kidneys and so on.

Should I stop Tresiba since it contains toxic substances?

You should not. First, you need it. The benefit of using it far outweighs not using it. You need to discuss with your doctor before you stop it. Second, I do recommend using the lowest dose possible. That is why I strongly urge you to eat right and exercise (for more information about treating diabetes, please read my other book about diabetes management<<Diabetes Questions and Answers More Than 400 Diabetes Frequently Asked Questions>>).

If I am allergic to Tresiba, what options do I have?

You can try other options, like Lantus, Basaglar, Levemir, or use fast-acting insulins like Humalog, Novolog, Fiasp, Apidra, or regular insulin using an insulin pump or V-go to deliver your insulin. If you are still allergic, then, you might have to try desensitization. Fortunately, I do not have any patients who needs to do that.

Chapter 6. NPH (Humulin N or Novolin N)

What is NPH (Humulin N or Novolin N)?

NPH stands for Neutral Protamine Hagedorn. Neutral refers to neutral pH (pH = 7), Protamine is a basic protein, and Hans Christian Hagedorn is an insulin researcher.

Lots of patients and doctors also shorten the name of this medication to N.

NPH insulin is made by mixing regular insulin (recombinant insulin made from bacteria or yeast) and protamine in exact proportions with zinc and phenol such that a neutral-pH is maintained and crystals form. Therefore, any insulin containing NPH could be cloudy, and you have to mix well before injection.

I have type 2 diabetes and my doctor started me on NPH (N). Should I give it in the morning or night?

NPH usually starts to work after one to two hours, then peaks after six to eight hours, It can last up to 24 hours. However, NPH has a significant peak. You have to take it at least two times a day. The usual recommendation is to take ⅔ of the daily dose in the morning and ⅓ of the daily dose at night. In this manner, the daytime peak falls at lunch time which can help control your lunch sugar from going up too high and not too low. Therefore it is very important that you do not miss your meal. Otherwise your sugar might go too low.

I sometimes recommend splitting it into three doses a day, every eight hours, for example 7am, 3pm, and 10-11 pm.

I have type 2 diabetes and my doctor wants to start me on NPH (N). What is the appropriate starting dose?

This actually depends on your sugar target, your sugar level, your weight, your kidney function, your liver function, and so on., However for a new insulin user, for elderly or thin patients, I usually start with 10 units in the morning and 5 units at night, for younger or more obese patients, I would start with 20-30 units in the morning and 10 units at night. Check your sugar at least three times a day. Based on your response to the insulin, you need to adjust the insulin dose accordingly. If your sugar is too low, you have to reduce your insulin dose right away. If your sugar is too high, I recommend you start adjusting after a week.

I have type 2 diabetes and my doctor wanted to start me on NPH (N). What is your recommendation for titrating the dose?

It is important to start on the right dose, but more important to titrate your dose based on your response. I want my patients to check sugar at least three times a day morning, lunch and bedtime, or at 7 am, 3pm and 10-11 pm, and stay on the same dose for 1 week if their sugar is not too low. I usually do not recommend having very tight control in the beginning to avoid hypoglycemia and to let patients become familiar with the regimen.

I ask patients to check their sugar 3 times a day. I adjust the morning dose based on before lunch sugar. If before lunch sugar is >140 mg/dl (your doctor might have different target for you) for two days, then increase by 2 units. I adjust the night dose based on bedtime and morning sugar. If both morning and bedtime sugar >140 mg/dl (your sugar target can be different), every two days you can increase by 2 units. I also give them a maximum dose like 40 units or 60 units based on their body size and other conditions like renal failure or liver failure.

It is very tricky to adjust NPH. Please review it with your physician.

Do you recommend vial or pen?

NPH comes in pen and vial. I recommend pen for most patients, but if your dose is very high, then vial is not a bad choice.

The U-100 of NPH is 100 units per ml. One 10 ml vial has 1000 units. One 3ml pen has 300 units.

If I am using the pen, can I leave the needle on for the next injection?

It is not recommended to leave the needle on for the next injection. It might increase the risk for inaccuracy and infection. It might also cause leaking. The needles are designed for single use. Reuse the needle can cause more injury to the injection site.

If I use the pen, should I leave the pen in the refrigerator or at room temperature?

After you start to use a new pen, you should leave it outside in a cool place, not exposed to the sun. You should not put it back in the refrigerator.

How long can I store the unopened pens and vials?

You need to store them at 36-46 F in the refrigerator. They should never be frozen. If frozen, you need to discard them. They can be stored until their expiration date.

How long can I store the unopened vial or pen at room temperature?

You should store unopened vials or pens of Humulin N in a refrigerator. If you do not have access to a refrigerator, the vial must be discarded after 31 days if stored at room temperature, below 86°F (30°C) . The pen must be discarded after 14 days if stored at room temperature, below 86°F (30°C) .

Novolin N vial lasts slightly longer, up to 42 days based on the company's released information.

How long can I store a vial or pen in use?

For a vial of Humulin N in use, you can store it in the refrigerator or at room temperature. You can use it for 31 days. In other words, you need to discard the vial even if there is still insulin in the vial after 31 days.

For a vial of Novolin N in use, you can store it in the refrigerator or at room temperature for 6 weeks (42 days).

For a pen in use, you need to store it at room temperature. Both Humulin N and Novolin N are the same for 14 days.

Please refer to the following table for storage for Humulin N.

	Unopened in refrigerator	Unopened at room temperature	Opened in use
Vial	Until expiration day	31 days	31 days
Pen	Until expiration day	14 days	14 days.

When in use a pen should not be put into a refrigerator.

How can I transport NPH insulin?

You can transport NPH as any other insulin, as you need them kept cool but not frozen. Based on availability and how long the journey, you can use different ways to keep your insulin cool. You can use bags, wallets, fridges with freezer packs, ice, or some fancy designed bags, and boxes.

However, if you are just on a short trip, and the temperature is below 86 F (30 C). You can transport pens either opened or unopened without special bags or boxes, or coolers. You can use either opened or unopened pens up to 14 days. You can use either opened or unopened vials up to 31 days.

I am using NPH and my morning sugar is still way too high. What should I do?

There are many reasons for your elevated sugar. The most common reasons for your high morning sugar are as follows:

- Ate too much at dinner and ate too late.

- Or ate something "wrong" at dinner like pizza.
- Not moving after your dinner.
- It is very tricky to titrate NPH. You might need to change to a different type of insulin.
- A week after you start your NPH insulin, you can start to titrate your dose. You can increase your dose by 2 units every two or three days if your morning sugar is still above your target, and your bedtime sugar is above 130-140.
- If you are taking NPH at dinner time, you can try to move your NPH to bedtime.
- There is a rare condition called Somogyi effect. Your sugar is too low at midnight and then rebounds too high in the morning. If this is the case which is suspected, you need to check your midnight or early morning sugar. If you have low sugar in the midnight or early morning, you apparently need to reduce your insulin. I recommend you reduce your insulin by half and continue to monitor your sugar and up titrate if needed.
- If possible, if you can have a CGM (continuous glucose monitor), this can be great tool for you.

I am using NPH and my morning sugar is too low. What should I do?

There are many reasons why you have low sugar. The most common reasons for your low morning sugars are as follows:

- You did not eat enough relative to your usual dinner portion.
- Did more exercise during the day compared to your usual days.
- Your kidney may be failing.
- If you are taking your NPH at bedtime, you might need to move to dinner time or afternoon around 3-4 pm.
- If you are taking your NPH at bed or dinner time, you might need to reduce your dose, or eat a small carb snack at bedtime if you are not overweight.

It is very difficult to adjust NPH doses as we discussed above. How much NPH to reduce if you have low sugar is dependent on many factors. If you are elderly and have heart disease or unstable kidney function, I would reduce by 50% if you have morning sugar below 70. If you are young but your morning sugar is below 50, you can consider to reduce your dose by 50% also.

I want to eat a big meal, so can I give more NPH?

NPH is an intermediate-acting insulin. It is really not ideal to use the intermediate-acting insulin to cover the meal. Overeating is not a good idea anyway.

Although after a single injection, it begins to work after 1-2 hours, NPH takes 4-6 hours to reach its peak. If your big feast is at lunch time, you might want to try increasing your morning NPH dose. The amount to increase is very hard to gauge. It certainly depends on how much you eat. I usually let people try to increase their dose by 30-50%. People usually eat 30-100% more on holidays. However, this practice is very tricky and can be dangerous. I really discourage you from overeating even during holidays.

I was hospitalized recently and the hospital used Lantus or Basaglar (or Levemir) on me, but I have NPH at home and am not able to afford any other insulin. What should I do?

Hospitals usually also have NPH in stock. However, your insulin might get changed for various reasons. If your insulin has been changed, it was most likely because you were not optimal while on NPH. Most likely your sugar was too low or fluctuated too much.

I recommend you switch to the hospital regimen if possible.

If you want to stay on NPH, you really need to discuss with your treating physician how to adjust your dose depending on your special situation.

My insurance changed my coverage. Now it doesn't pay for any Lantus or Basaglar, Tresiba, Toujeo or Levemir. What can I do?

You might have to use NPH (N), either Humulin N or Novolin N. Now Novolin N is more affordable. It costs $ 26 dollars per 1000 units (10 ml vial) at Wal-Mart or Sam's club. You can try ⅔ of your total basal insulin dose before breakfast, and ⅓ before dinner.

Then you can adjust your morning dose based on before lunch sugar and dinner dose based on bedtime and morning sugars. You can increase your dose by 2 units if your sugar is above your preset target for consecutive two days; you can reduce by 2 units or more if you sugar is below your preset target. It is very tricky to adjust NPH. You need more instructions from your physician.

Can I mix my NPH with regular insulin?

Yes, you can. However, if your total insulin dose is less than 20 units, I do not recommend doing that. When the dose is less than 20 units, the percentage of error is too high and the procedure is complicated.

How do I mix my NPH and regular insulin or other short-acting insulin?

It can be very tricky. If you have shaky hands, or vision issues, I recommend not trying it.

Here are steps to mix NPH and fast-acting insulin:

1. Clean the area where you will work with your insulin.

2. Gather everything you need, such as your NPH, your regular insulin, alcohol swabs, insulin pen (large enough to hold both NPH and regular insulin R), sharps container, and two pieces of paper to write down your insulin dose.

3. Check the drug labels to be sure of what they are. Check the expiration date on the vials and the date you opened it (started to use it). If your total daily NPH dose is less than 30, I recommend writing down the new expiration date, which is a month from the day of starting the bottle. Do not use a drug that is past the expiration date.

4. Look at the insulin.

5. Most insulin is clear (for instance, regular insulin, Humalog, Novolog, Apidra should always appear clear). Do not use the insulin if the drug appears to have pieces in it or if it is discolored.

6. NPH is cloudy, but should not have clumps inside. If you see any discoloration or clumps in the bottle, you need to discard it.

7. Mix NPH well. To do this, you need to roll the vial between your hands 20 times, and then also turn it gently from side to side 20 times. Do not shake it.

8. Get two pieces of paper and write down the units for NPH and total units of NPH+ clear insulin on one piece of paper, make a circle around the total insulin units to distinguish from the NPH units. Write down the units for clear insulin dose on the other piece of paper, and put the clear insulin on the paper.

9. Remove the lids from the top of the insulin vials. (After the lids are removed, they will not go back onto the vial. The rubber tops will provide a seal.) Wipe the rubber tops with an alcohol swab or a cotton ball moistened with alcohol.

10. Remove the plastic needle cap by pulling it straight off. Do not touch the needle. If the needle touches any surface, you have to change it.

11. Pull back the plunger of the syringe to the number of units of insulin you must take from the cloudy insulin bottle (you already wrote on the paper). This will pull air into the syringe.

12. Place the vial of cloudy insulin on a flat surface, and push the needle through the rubber top. Push down on the plunger to push air into the vial. Do not pull insulin into the syringe at this time. Take the needle out of the bottle.

13. Using the same syringe, pull back the plunger to the number of units of insulin you want from the clear insulin bottle (you already wrote down on the paper). This will pull air into the syringe.

14. Place the vial of clear insulin on a flat surface, and push the needle through the rubber top. Push down on the plunger to push air into the vial. Leave the needle in the bottle.

15. Turn the clear insulin vial and syringe upside down, holding the syringe and needle in place.

16. Make sure the tip of the insulin needle is in the insulin solution. Then pull the plunger back by the flat knob. This will draw insulin into the syringe. Keep pulling slowly on the knob until the insulin reaches the number on the paper for clear insulin.

17. Check for air bubbles in the syringe. This is important. Having air space instead of insulin may lead to an incorrect dose.

18. Using the same syringe, carefully insert the needle into the cloudy bottle. Be sure not to push any of the insulin from the syringe into the bottle.

19. Turn the cloudy insulin vial and syringe upside down, holding the syringe and needle in place.
20. Make sure the tip of the insulin needle is in the insulin solution. Then pull the plunger back by the flat knob, slowly until it reaches the total units (we put down on the paper with the circle). Be careful not to pull any air into the syringe or pass the total units.
21. It is important not to pull past the total number of units. Once the insulins are mixed in the syringe, you cannot push any of the insulin back into the second bottle. And you cannot get rid of the extra amount in any way.
22. If you draw too much insulin, throw away the syringe and start over with a new one.
23. Remove the needle from the vial.
24. Now you can give the shot.

Can I mix any other insulin with NPH?

You can mix Humalog, Novolog or Apidra with NPH. As above, you want to draw clear insulin into the syringe first then drawn NPH. Again, I really discourage this practice. It is so much easier just to give two shots.

What else is in NPH?

For humulin N, each milliliter of Humulin N contains 100 units of insulin (human), 0.35 mg of protamine sulfate, 16 mg of glycerin, 3.78 mg of dibasic sodium phosphate, 1.6 mg of metacresol, 0.65 mg of phenol, zinc oxide content adjusted to provide 0.025 mg zinc ion, and water for injection.

Novolin N has similar contents.

What is metacresol (m-cresol)? Is it toxic?

It is a derivative of phenol and is an isomer of p-cresol and o-crestol. Together with many other compounds, m-cresol is traditionally extracted from coal tar.

The synonyms are: 1-Hydroxy-3-methylbenzene; 3-Cresol; 3-Hydroxytoluene; 3-Methylphenol; m-Cresole; m-Cresylic acid; m-Hydroxytoluene; m-Kresol; m-Methylphenol; m-Oxytoluene; m-Toluol; phenol, 3-methyl; Metacresol.

It is used as a preservative. It is certainly toxic. Some patients' adverse reactions to NPH might be related to reaction to m-cresol. Skin inflammation is characterized by itching, scaling, reddening, or occasionally blistering.

It might be carcinogenic, meaning it might cause cancer. It might also cause damage to your central nervous system (brain and spinal cord), liver, kidneys and so on if consumed enough.

Should I stop NPH since it contains toxic substances?

You should not. First, you need it. The benefit of using it far outweighs not using it. You need to discuss with your doctor before you stop it; Second, I recommend using the lowest dose possible. That is why I strongly urge you to eat right and exercise. (For more information about treat diabetes, please read my other book about diabetes management <<Diabetes Questions and Answers More Than 400 Diabetes Frequently Asked Questions>>.)

If I am allergic to NPH, what options do I have?

You can try Lantus, Basaglar, Levemir, Tresiba or use fast-acting insulins like Humalog, Novolog, Apidra, Fiasp or regular insulin using an insulin pump or V-go to deliver your insulin. If you are still allergic, you might have to desensitize. Fortunately, I do not have any patients who need to do that.

I am traveling and I ran out of my prescription. What can I do?

You can buy Novolin N from Wal-Mart for $26 (Novolin N) without a prescription. It is over-the-counter. You might need a coupon for this price.

I have type 1 diabetes, and I have severe fluctuating sugar. What should I do?

If you have type 1 diabetes, you should not be on NPH. type 1 diabetes is very tricky already and using NPH only makes it trickier. For most type 1 diabetes, sugar can never be controlled with NPH. You need to demand your insurance company to cover other insulins.

I have type 2 diabetes. Can you give me some guidelines on adjusting my dose of NPH?

Usually you have to take NPH two or three times a day.

For twice day schedule, one dose before breakfast, and one dose before dinner or at bedtime.

For three times a day, I usually set up a every 8 hours schedule. I usually give my patients a specific time like 7am. 3pm and 11 pm.

First, you need to have a target that you have discussed with your physician. This is important. Otherwise how will you know if your sugar is too high or too low? The target is usually decided by your tendency to get low sugar, your age, your general health, your liver and kidney conditions.

If you are taking NPH two or three times a day, you need to check your sugar three to four times a day.

For reasonably healthy patients who do not get low sugar easily, I recommend these targets for you:

1. Morning sugar is 100-130, but occasionally 70-99 is okay.
2. Before lunch sugar is 100-130, but occasionally 70-99 is okay.
3. Before dinner sugar is 100-130, but occasionally 70-99 is okay.
4. 9 pm sugar is 130-160, but occasionally 100-129 is okay.

Adjust morning dose based on morning and lunch sugars.

> If morning sugar is in the target or above the target range, then look at previous 2 days sugar at lunch time,
>   o If lunchtime sugar is in the target, keep the same dose.
>   o If lunchtime sugar is over the target, increase by 2 units every two days
>   o If lunchtime sugar is below the target, decrease by 2 units every two days
> If morning sugar is below the target, you need to decrease the dose, regardless of lunchtime sugar. Sometimes, it can be a hard decision, if your sugar is 70-99, and you are going to eat, you can keep the same dose to see. If your sugar is 50-69 mg/dl, you can try to decrease by 50%, if it is very low-- below 50, you might omit one dose completely.

If you are taking another dose at dinner time. Dinner time dose is adjusted based on the bedtime sugar and/or previous days' morning sugar.

> If dinner time sugar is in the normal range or above the normal, and previous days' bedtime and morning are in the normal range, then keep the same dose.
>

➤ If dinner time sugar is in the normal range or above the normal, and previous days' bedtime and morning are above the normal range for two consecutive days, then increase the dinner time NPH by 2 units. I usually set up a maximum dose of 60-80 units.

➤ If dinner time sugar is below the normal range, if <49 mg/dl, you might have to completely hold the dose, and eat your dinner. If 50-69 mg/dl, you can consider giving half the dose and eat dinner. Certainly, you always need to check your sugar.

If you are also taking NPH at bedtime, then you adjust the dose based on previous morning sugar. Certainly if you sugar is low already at bedtime, then you need to reduce the dose, eat a snack or omit the dose completely.

What you proposed above is too complicated. I tried it, my sugar is still up and down. What can I do?

It is very difficult to use NPH. Sugar level is expected to fluctuate. Besides insulin, sugar is determined by not just what you eat, how much you eat, how much exercise you get, but it also is determined by your emotional status (too much stress) or any pain. Lots of other medications also can affect your sugar.

So if you see your sugar is not the same every time, it is normal.

If you have trouble adjusting your insulin dose, please observe the following:

Keep your sugar target in mind. You know your sugar target so you know your sugar is too high or too low. You might need to have a different target. Discuss with your doctor.

Shunzhong Shawn Bao, MD

If you are relatively healthy and not prone to having hypoglycemia

> If insulin dosing time sugar is >70, you can give the full dose and eat your meal.
> If insulin dosing time sugar is between 50-69, you can try giving half of the dose and eat your meal.

> If insulin dosing time sugar is <49, you can omit the dose and eat your meal.

Again, based on your history of hypoglycemia or other commodities (heart disease, liver disease, kidney disease), your doctor might set your target differently. Based on your situation, your doctor might set a target of 100 mg/dl

> If insulin dosing time sugar is >100, you can give the full dose and eat your meal.
> If insulin dosing time sugar is between 70-100, you can give half of the dose and eat your meal.
> If insulin dosing time sugar is <70, you should omit the dose and eat your meal.

It is very important for you to check your sugar and write down what you did, and bring the log to your doctor. She or he will make recommendations based on your specific situation.

Another option is that you can keep the same dose every day. If your sugar is below the target and not at meal time, you need to eat a snack and check your sugar to make sure to be back above the target.

Chapter 7. Humulin R U-500

What is U-500 insulin?

U-500 insulin is manufactured regular human insulin and is 5x as concentrated. In the old days, it was pig insulin. It starts to works between 30 and to 60 minutes after injection, peaks after three to five hours and last up to 12 hours or longer. It starts to work slightly slower than regular insulin, but runs as long as NPH.

When do we use U-500?

Usually we use it if your total insulin needs are more than 200 units. I personally do not believe in using high dose insulin. Currently I only have 2 patients on U-500, whom I inherited from retired colleague.

Who are the typical patients currently treated with U-500?

The most common patients have uncontrolled diet and are morbidly obese; there are some patients with lipodystrophy (could be due to a gene mutation or drugs like protease inhibitors for human immunodeficiency).

Why do you avoid prescribing U-500?

Here are the reasons.

1. I think most patients do not really need so high a dose of insulin. Most patients really need more diet and lifestyle

education. Their need for insulin will drastically decreas after diet control and a little more exercise.

2. The dose is so high that it might cause unstable sugar which makes patients eat more to prevent hypoglycemia which will cause patients to eat even more.

3. The U-500 dosing is very confusing to the patients and pharmacist. Due to miscommunication among the physician, patient, and pharmacist, serious mistakes have been made which have led to death. The confusion is mainly from the units and volume. Even to this day, the ADA (American Diabetes Association) website is still wrong about U-500. It says, *"This means that every 1 unit of U-500 is the same as 5 units of your usual insulin."* *(http://clinical.diabetesjournals.org/content/30/2/86).* This is wrong. 1 unit of U-500 is 1 unit. U-500 is just 5 times as concentrated as regular insulin. It just has less volume. If it were administered in the same volume, then you would have 5 times as much insulin as in regular U-100. You might still be confused. You are not alone. Do not worry, even professionals from the ADA made the mistake, as above. Luckily, now we have the U-500 pen. You just use it like any other pen. You need no conversions and do not have a chance to make mistake. However, there are doctors who are still making the mistake. They are writing five times less insulin because they think U-500 is five times more powerful.

4. Nowadays, we have more options like U-300 of Toujeo, and U-200 Tresiba.

5. Most importantly, we have more options to treat severe insulin resistant patients, especially those unable to get a controlled diet , and patients with GLP-1 agonist and SGLT2 antagonists.

6. Finally, I do not believe the more the better when considering insulin. As we can see, insulin does have side effects. You need to strive to get your lowest dose possible.

Do I need to do some conversion with U-500 insulin pen?

The good news for the pen is that you do not need to do any conversions. You just use it as you would any other pen.

Doctors write their prescriptions like for other insulin, just writing how many units to give. You do not even have to think about U-500, or U-100. The doctor only needs to think about how many units to give.

I was prescribed U-500 vial and tuberculin syringes. However, I could not get tuberculin syringes. What can I do?

You need to talk to your prescribing physician to see if your prescription can be changed to the U-500 pen. Then you can use the pen as any other insulin pen.

If your insurance only pays for the vial, then you need to go back to your physician to see if a new prescription can be written using U-500 insulin syringe. Now BD makes a specialized insulin syringe for U-500. I strongly recommended using this specialized insulin syringe to avoid any error. If you use this special U-500 syringe, you do not need to do any conversion.

However, if you cannot get your U-500 syringe and you have to use a U-100 syringe, a prescription might look like the following:

Humulin R U-500 80 units (16 units mark using U-100 syringe) sc one hour before breakfast; 80 units (16 units mark using U-100 syringe) sc one hour before lunch and 40 units (8 units mark using U-100 syringe) sc one hour before dinner.

Can I use U-500 in an insulin pump?

There are successful reports of using insulin pumps but again, I do not like this idea. U-500 is more like an intermediate insulin. Using a pump, we mainly just give basal insulin. Again as we discussed before, in terms of insulin, I do not think the more the better. You need to strive to get your insulin dose down.

Can I mix U-500 and U-100 insulin and do one injection?

No, it has not been recommended. I do not recommend it either. However, there are patients who are using it.

How long can I store U-500 insulin?

Unused vials or pens can be stored in the refrigerator until the expiration date. After opening a vial, you can use it for up to 40 days. It can be stored either in the refrigerator or at room temperature. After 40 days, any remaining insulin in the vial should be thrown away.

Store opened (in-use) Humulin R U-500 KwikPens at room temperature for up to 28 days. Do not refrigerate opened KwikPens. Throw away any opened KwikPen after 28 days of use, even if there is insulin left in the pen.

What else is in U-500 human insulin?

Humulin R U-500 is a sterile, aqueous, and colorless solution. Humulin R U-500 contains 500 units of insulin in each milliliter. Each milliliter of Humulin R U-500 also contains glycerin 16 mg, metacresol 2.5 mg, zinc oxide to supplement the endogenous zinc to obtain a total zinc content of 0.017 mg/100 units, and water for injection.

What is m-cresol? Is it toxic?

It is a derivative of phenol and is an isomer of p-cresol and o-cresol. Together with many other compounds, m-cresol is traditionally extracted from coal tar.

The synonyms are: 1-Hydroxy-3-methylbenzene; 3-Cresol; 3-Hydroxytoluene; 3-Methylphenol; m-Cresole; m-Cresylic acid; m-Hydroxytoluene; m-Kresol; m-Methylphenol; m-Oxytoluene; m-Toluol; phenol, 3-methyl, Metacresol.

It is used as a preservative. It is certainly toxic. Some patients' adverse reactions to U-500 might be related to a reaction to m-cresol. Skin inflammation is characterized by itching, scaling, reddening, or occasionally blistering.

It might be carcinogenic, meaning it might cause cancer. It might also cause damage to your central nervous system (brain and spinal cord), liver, kidneys and so on if you get enough.

Should I stop U-500 since it contains toxic substance?

Unfortunately all currently used insulin have toxic substances. This is why I recommend my patients strive to optimize their diet and exercise and in combination with other medications to use minimal dose of insulin possible.

How can I titrate my U-500 insulin dose?

It can be very complicated. You'd better talk to your prescribing physician.

Your dose actually is determined by previous days' responses which is very difficult to explain.

You can try the following strategy, as a simple sliding scale. You might want to ask your doctor for a more detailed sliding scale, just for you.

> ➤ If your dosing time sugar is>100, give the scheduled dose.
> ➤ If your dosing time sugar is between 70 and 99, give half of the scheduled dose.
> ➤ If your dosing time sugar is <70, hold your dose.

Chapter 8. Inhaled insulin

What is inhaled insulin?

Afrezza is the only inhaled form of insulin. It is rapid-acting. It is used for premeal insulin.

Who can use it?

Afrezza is indicated for both type 1 and type 2 diabetes to control mealtime sugar. Both type 1 and type 2 diabetes patients without contraindication for Afrezza can use it.

Who cannot use it?

Anybody:

> Is a smoker
> Has chronic or active lung disease
> Has asthma/COPD/interstitial lung disease
> Has shortness of breath
> Has history of any anaphylaxis. Anaphylaxis is a life threatening allergic reaction characterized by difficulty in breathing, a sudden drop of blood pressure, etc.
> Has strong family history of lung cancer or personal history of lung cancer.
> Failed a lung function test, indicating lung disease.

What is the advantage of using Afrezza?

- ➤ It is convenient. Before the meal, you can just inhale. It is more acceptable in public in case you use it in public.
- ➤ No needles. It is estimated as high as 20% of people have trypanophobia (extremely afraid of needles).
- ➤ The hypoglycemia rate may be lower, since the insulin is being absorbed quickly and being cleared quickly.
- ➤ Storage temperature excursion is permitted up to 86 F (30 C).

How should Afrezza be stored?

Unopened foil sealed package can be stored in the refrigerator until expiration date.

If stored at room temperature (temperature excursion is allowed up to 86 F), Afrezza should be used in 10 days.

Opened strips can be stored at room temperature or in the refrigerator for up to three days. If stored in a refrigerator, it needs to get back to room temperature before using.

What is the dosage form?

It comes in a single use cartridge of 4 units and 8 units. In other words, the minimal dosage increment is 4 units.

What is the common adverse reaction?

The most common adverse reactions are: low sugar, cough, throat irritation, or pain.

What are the warnings and precautions?

- ➤ Acute bronchospasm
- ➤ At the time of changing regimen, you might experience too high or too low sugar
- ➤ Hypoglycemia (low sugar)
- ➤

➤ Lung function might decrease. Although it is believed that this is not clinically significant, it is required to have a lung function test before starting Afrezza, after six months, and yearly thereafter.
➤ Afrezza should not be used in patients with active lung cancer. I also don't recommend use in patients with personal or family history of lung cancer or smoking.

➤ Hypersensitivity can occur with any medication including Afrezza and can be life threatening.
➤ All potential side effects of insulin can occur to Afrezza, like low potassium, weight gain, or fluid retention.

I have never been on premeal insulin. At what dose should I start?

You can start at the lowest dose like the 4 unit cartridge (blue). After you are stabilized, you can start to titrate.

I have been taking premeal insulin. How do I convert?

Since Afrezza only comes in the dose form of 4 units increment, sometime, you have to use approximations. Most of the time, it is recommended to do a 1 unit to 1 unit conversion.

I recommend starting low and then titrating. For example, if you were taking 10 units of premeal insulin, you can try the Afrezza 8 unit cartridge (green).

How do I titrate on Afrezza dose?

You first need to set up your target. You need to work with your doctor to decide what the best target is for you. This is mainly determined by your propensity to develop low sugar. This is affected by your body weight, your liver and kidney function, and your comorbidities. The actual daily dose is also determined by what, how much and how you consume your meal, and your pre and post meal activity. Lots of other issues can also affect your insulin needs.

You need to check your sugar before each meal and at bedtime. I recommend adjusting your next day's premeal based on previous day's response. Again, adjusting insulin dosage is always very tricky. You need to consider your activity level, what you eat, and how you eat. Generally speaking, you can adjust your morning dose based on previous pre-lunch sugar, your lunch dose based on previous pre-dinner sugar, pre-dinner dose based on previous bedtime sugar. If sugar has not come down to your target range, I suggest increasing by 4 units. After your sugar is stabilized, titrate again.

What is the maximum dose?

The maximum dose is 24 units (three cartridge of 8 units).

Do I need a pen to be prepared just in case?

I think this is a really good idea. If it's not possible to get a sample, you will need a prescription for it. You can give it to yourself when you have a respiratory infection or any circumstances or when you need more than 24 units of insulin.

When should I temporarily hold my Afrezza?

➢ When your sugar is too low.
➢ When you are having a respiratory system infection.
➢ You are developing DKA (diabetic ketoacidosis).
➢ When your sugar is too high and it cannot be controlled by Afrezza, you need to go to the ER or your doctor's office right way.

Chapter 9. Long-acting insulin and GLP-1 agonist combination

-SOLIQUA 100/33

-XULTOPHY® 100/3.6

What is Soliqua 100/33?

Soliqua 100/33 is a combination of long-acting insulin glargine and GLP-1 agonist lixisenatide.

What is glargine?

Glargine is a long-acting analog, usually used as basal insulin. See section Lantus or Basaglar.

What is GLP-1 agonist?

A group of gut hormones called incretins are secreted from the gut. This group of hormones regulates insulin secretion and gut mobility. One incretin is glucagon like peptide-1 (GLP-1). However, the endogenous GLP-1 is very short lived, only lasts a few seconds. Medications like lixisenatide (Adlyxin) or liraglutide (Victoza) are engineered and will last much longer. They restore incretin-based insulin secretion and modulate gut motility.

What does the 100/33 following Soliqua mean?

100/33 means 100 units of glargine in one milliliter; 33 means 33 ug of lixisenatide in one milliliter. The minimal dose of Soliqua 100/33 is 15 units (15 units of glargine and 5 ug of lixisenatide).
If you use 20 units, you will get 20 units of glargine and 6.67 ug of lixisenatide.
If you use 60 units (which is the maximum dose allowed), you will get 60 units of glargine and 20 ug of lixisenatide.

Is lixisenatide also available by itself?

Lixisenatide is also available under the brand-name of Adlyxin. I, personally, have never prescribed it.

What is Xultophy 100/3.6?

Xultophy 100/3.6 is the combination of long-acting insulin Tresiba (degludec) and Victoza (liraglutide).

What does the number 100/3.6 mean after Xultophy?

100/3.6 means there is 100 units of Tresiba in one milliliter and 3.6 mg of Victoza.

The recommended starting dose is 16 units (16 units of Tresiba and 0.58 mg of Victoza), but you can start with 10 units (10 units of Tresiba and 0.36 mg of Victoza) and work up.

The maximum dose allowed is 50 units (50 units of Tresiba and 1.8 mg of Victoza).

What is the benefit of using GLP-1 agonist in diabetics?

GLP-1 agonists are now very popular in diabetes management. They were found to have the following benefits:

1) Reduce A1c very effectively. They can reduce A1c by over 1% depending on the starting point.
2) Help control appetite and slow down the gastric emptying, therefore it can help you lose 3-10% of your body weight (depending on different clinical trials).
3) In some clinical trials, GLP-1 agonists-treated group had lower rates of cardiovascular events and death from any cause than did those in the control group.

Why do we use a combination of long-acting insulin and a GLP-1 agonist?

1. Basal insulin (long-acting) mainly controls fasting blood sugar.
2. Incretin based GLP-1 mainly controls post-prandial (after meal) sugar.
3. Basal insulin can let beta cells "rest" and "work" when they need to.
4. GLP-1 agonist also reduces appetite and slows gastric intestinal motility, therefore sugar can become more stabilized.
5. Insulin causes weight gain, while GLP-1 can reduce insulin needs and cause weight loss. So the weight gain can be mitigated while sugar is better controlled.
6. Combination of two medications in one shot, so you can have one shot instead of two.

What is the disadvantage of taking the combination?

You cannot adjust each individual component. If for the reasons we mentioned that you are unable to take one of the components, then both components will be stopped.

I have a patient who was on Lantus. Her sugar needed to be better controlled; I switched her to Soliqua 100/33. She was doing very well on Soliqua, but her insurance refused to pay.

After she finished the samples I gave her, she was not back to Lantus. Her sugar went over 500, and she had to go to the ER. Therefore, if for some reason you do not have the combination, you can continue the insulin you had before and let your physician know.

What else in Soliqua 100/33 besides glargine and lixisenatide?

Each Soliqua 100/33 prefilled single-patient disposable pen contains 300 units of insulin glargine and 100 ug of lixisenatide in a 3 mL clear, almost colorless, sterile, and aqueous solution. Soliqua 100/33 contains the following inactive ingredients (per mL): 3 mg of methionine, 2.7 mg of metacresol, 20 mg of glycerol, 30 mcg of zinc, hydrochloric acid, sodium hydroxide and water for injection as inactive ingredients.

Who should not take the combination long-acting insulin and GLP-1 agonists?

1. You should not have any history of hypersensitivity to any component of Soliqua 100/33 or Xultophy 100/3.6.
2. You should not take it if you have a history of pancreatitis.
3. You should not take it if you have family with pancreatic cancer.
4. You should not take it if you have triglycerides over 1000 that are not controlled.
5. You should not take it if you have a history of medullary thyroid cancer or (MEN II)- very rare.
6. You should not take it if you have severe uncontrolled gastroparesis.
7. You should not take it if you have severe nausea or vomiting.
8. You should not take it if you have very severe renal dysfunction (discuss with your treating physician) especially if you are taking Soliqua 100/33. Xultophy 100/3.6 is okay with most patients.

9. If your doctor decides you need more insulin to control your sugar and you are using the maximum dose of the combinations already.
10. If you are pregnant, planning to get pregnant, or nursing a baby, you should not take the combination.
11. Certainly, if your sugar is low already.

When should I temporarily hold or permanently stop Soliqua 100/33 or Xultophy 100/3.6?

If you develop any of the following, you need to stop and talk to your physician:

1. If you develop or suspect you have hypersensitivity to any component of Soliqua 100/33 or Xultophy100/3.6.
2. If you suspect you have pancreatitis (symptoms: severe nausea, vomiting, and abdominal pain radiating to your back).
3. If you have a family member diagnosed with pancreatic cancer.
4. If you have triglycerides over 1000 that are not controlled.
5. If you are diagnosed with medullary thyroid cancer or (MEN II)- very rare.
6. If you develop severe nausea and/or vomiting and are suspected to have severe uncontrolled gastroparesis.
7. If you are developing severe renal dysfunction (discuss with your treating physician) especially if you are taking Soliqua 100/33.
8. If your doctor decides you need more insulin to control your sugar, and you are already using the maximum dose of the combinations. In this situation, I would rather prescribed insulin and GLP-1 agonist separately and then I can adjust the dose separately.
9. If you are pregnant, planning to get pregnant, or nursing a baby, you should not take the combination.

What are other possible adverse side effects?

As we discussed, Soliqua 100/33 and Xultophy 100/3.6 are insulin and GLP-1 agonists, so they might have the adverse effects of both medications, like hypoglycemia, hypokalemia, weight gain, water retention and so on.

When should I take it?

1. I recommend you take it at least 30-60 minutes before your first meal every day.
2. Antibiotics, acetaminophen, or other medications that are particularly dependent on threshold concentrations for efficacy or for which a delay in effect is undesirable, should be administered at least 1 hour before Soliqua 100/33 injection or Xultophy 100/3.6.
3. If you are taking daily oral contraceptives, it should be taken at least one hour before Soliqua 100/33 or Xultophys 100/3.6 administration or 11 hours after.

What can I do if I miss my dose?

It can be tricky. This is from my experience but not FDA approved.

The standard recommendation is to not give an extra dose and not increase your next dose.

For Soliqua 100/33, if you realized it before lunch, you might try to give it. If you are prone to having low sugar at night, then you need to cut down your dose by 20%. If you miss your dose and don't realize it until 7 pm, you can give as soon as possible , but reduce your next scheduled dose by 50%. If your dose is less than 30 units, you cannot reduce by 50% since the minimal dose it 15 units. In this case, you might just miss one dose.

For Xultophy, if you miss a dose, you have following four options:

1. You can give a catch up dose as long as your next dose is 12 hours away.
2. If your next dose is within 12 hours, you can give a dose as soon as possible and then give next dose after 12 hours and then back to your normal schedule.
3. If your next dose is within 12 hours, one option is to just miss a dose.
4. If your next dose is within 12 hours, you can still give your full dose as soon as possible. For next dose, you can reduce by 50% at regular time and then back to regular dose and regular time.

How should I store Soliqua 100/33 or Xultophy 100/3.6?

Unopened Soliqua and Xultophy should be refrigerated (36-46 F) until their expiration date. If ever frozen, you need to throw them away.

After the first use, store them at room temperature below 86°F (30°C). Replace the pen cap after each use to protect from light.

For Soliqua 100/33, discard the pen 14 days after first use (even if there is product left).

For Xultophy 100/3.6, discard the pen 21 days after the first use(even if there is product left).

Always remove the needle after each injection and store the Soliqua 100/33 pen without a needle attached. This prevents contamination and/or infection, or leakage of the Soliqua 100/33 pen, and will ensure accurate dosing. Always use a new needle for each injection to prevent contamination.

Shunzhong Shawn Bao, MD

How can I adjust my doses of Soliqua 100/33?

I usually recommend patients start at the lowest dose possible and follow my diet recommendations as much as they can. I want my patients to stay on the lowest dose for a week and then to adjust their doses after.

For Soliqua 100/33, the minimum dose is 15 units (15 units of glargine and 5 ug of lixisenatide). I recommend patients stay on this dose for one week.

Check sugar twice a day, morning and bedtime. Set a target for them. The target should be individualized depending on patient's age, liver function, renal function, history of hypoglycemia, and other cardiovascular comorbidities.

For young and relatively healthy patients, my target for them is morning 100 mg/dl and night 130-140 mg/dl

For patients with a moderate risk for hypoglycemia, my target for them is morning 130 mg/dl and night 160 mg/dl.

For patients with a high risk for hypoglycemia, my target for them is morning 160 mg/dl and night 200 mg/dl.

After one week, if their sugar has not reached target, I would increase the dose by two units every two days. Do not increase the dose if either morning or night has reached its goal.

Any time your sugar falls below 100 mg/dl, I would recommend reducing the dose by 2 units. Sometimes, I let patients stay the same dose if sugar above 80. Again, the targets need individualized. Please refer to Chapter 1.

If your morning sugar (your dosing time sugar) is below the target, then you need to reduce your dose based on your target and how low the sugar is.

How can I adjust my dose of Xultophy 100/3.6?

I usually recommend patients start at the lowest dose possible and follow my diet recommendations as much as they can. I want my patient to stay on the lowest dose for a week and then to adjust their doses.

For Xultophy 100/3.6, the minimal starting dose is 16 units (16 units of Tresiba and 0.58 mg of Victoza). Same thing, I would recommend my patients staying on this dose for one week.

Check sugar twice a day, morning and bedtime. Set a target for them. The target should be individualized depending on patient's age, liver function, renal function, history of hypoglycemia, and other cardiovascular comorbidities.

For young and healthy patients, my target for them is morning 100 mg/dl and night 130-140 mg/dl.

For patients with a moderate risk for hypoglycemia, my target for them is morning 130 mg/dl and night 160 mg/dl.

For patients with a high risk for hypoglycemia, my target for them is morning 160 mg/dl and night 200 mg/dl.

After one week, if your sugar has not reached its target, I would increase the dose by 2 units **every three days**. Do not increase the dose if either morning or night sugar reached its goal.

Any time your sugar falls below 100 or your specified target, I would recommend reducing the dose by 2 units. If falls below 70, I recommend to reduce by 50%.

What should I do if I use the maximum dose, but my sugar is still high?

You should discuss this with your physician. You need add-on therapy. I heard someone say to double the dose or add another shot of glargine (Lantus, Basaglar, Toujeo) or Tresiba. I do not recommend doing this. It can be dangerous and confusing.

Chapter 10. Fast-acting insulin analogs

Types:

Humalog-lispro

Novolog-aspart

Apidra-glulisine

Fisap-aspart+niacinamide

What is Humalog?

Humalog is a rapid-acting human insulin analog-lispro produced by bacteria. It is usually used for pre-meal insulin, sliding scale (correction), and emergency use. It can be used in type 1, type 2, and gestational diabetes.

What are the dose forms for Humalog?

Humalog 100 units/mL (U-100) is available as 10 mL vials or 3 mL vials

Humalog KwikPen® (prefilled) 3ml • Humalog® Junior KwikPen® (prefilled) 3ml •cartridges 3 mL

Humalog 200 units/mL (U-200) is available as • 3 mL Humalog KwikPen® (prefilled)

How fast? How long does it work after being subcutaneously injected?

Humalog is a rapid-acting insulin. In most patients, it starts to work after ~15-20 minutes, has its peak effect after 60-90 minutes, and can last 4-5 hours. Its effect on different patients can vary drastically. Even in the same patient, it can be different day to day.

What else is in Humalog?

Humalog is a clear, colorless solution. Each milliliter of Humalog U-100 contains insulin lispro 100 units, 16 mg glycerin, 1.88 mg dibasic sodium phosphate, 3.15 mg metacresol, zinc oxide content adjusted to provide 0.0197 mg zinc ion, trace amounts of phenol, and water for injection. Insulin lispro has a pH of 7.0 to 7.8. The pH is adjusted by addition of aqueous solutions of hydrochloric acid 10% and/or sodium hydroxide 10%.

Each milliliter of Humalog U-200 contains insulin lispro 200 units, 16 mg glycerin, 5 mg tromethamine, 3.15 mg metacresol, zinc oxide content adjusted to provide 0.046 mg zinc ion, trace amounts of phenol, and water for Injection.

What is the difference between Humalog U-100 and U-200?

To you, you can say there is no difference. As you can see above, U-200 has 200 units in 1 ml of solution, but you work in terms of units and U-200 only comes as a pen which only marks in units. Therefore, for most patients, you do not need to worry. However, you should never get insulin from a U-200 pen and use it for different purposes. So far, I have no patients doing that.

As said above, Humalog U-200 has twice the amount of units in 1ml insulin. The U-200 pen has 600 units instead of 300 units that are in the U-100 pen.

Who should consider the Humalog U-200 pen?

- ➢ Someone who is using more than 15 units for pre-meal insulin.
- ➢ Someone who finishes more than four pens (especially more than five) each month.

I was switched from Humalog U-100 to U-200. Do I need any conversion factor?

Humalog U-100 to U-200 has a 1 unit to 1 unit conversion. When you use the pen, just use it as any other pen. The only thing you need to focus on is how many units.

Why do I need Humalog U-200?

Well, if you are using a high dose of insulin, then the U-200 can last twice as long. For some patients, they might also save money since companies usually run some promotions for new products.

I think Humalog U-200 might have the following advantages (not all proven). I just have these educated guesses:

- ➢ U-200 has half the volume, so the injury to the injection site will be smaller.
- ➢ U-200 has half the toxins like metacresol. This chemical might contribute to scar formation or lipodystrophy at the injection site. As we know, this chemical is also toxic to central nervous system and cause cancer, although we

do not know how much damage it can cause with the level in your insulin injection. The less is the better.

What should I do if I overdose myself with fast-acting insulin?

This happens often. I repeat myself here.

Humalog, Novolog, Apidra, Novolin R, Humulin R and Fiasp are fast-acting insulins. As we discussed above, we usually use them as premeal insulin or correction (sliding scale) to get sugar down fast. In other words, it can get your sugar down starting after 15-30 minutes and peaks after 60-120 minutes. It can last 4-5 hours. In patients with kidney dysfunction or liver dysfunction, it even can last much longer.

Here is what you should do:

> ➤ Calm down and write down how much insulin you have overdosed.
> ➤ If you have an insulin carb ratio, then calculate how many carbs you need to eat. For example, if your insulin carb ratio is 1:8 and if you overdose yourself by 5 units, you need to eat 5x8=40 g of carbs.
> ➤ If you do not have an insulin carb ratio, but with a fixed dose before meals, calculate the portion of the overdosed insulin to your meal insulin. For example, if you give 12 units for your balanced meal and you overdose 3 units, you need to eat one quarter (3/12=¼) of your regular balanced meal.
> ➤ Certainly you need to check your sugar more often the next 5 hours or before next meal.
> ➤ You need to be vigilant until your sugar is stabilized.
> ➤ It is also a good idea to tell your family or friends what happened, and they can be vigilant also.
> ➤ Always be prepared. Always have some carbs with you.

➤ If you have type 1 diabetes or unstable sugar, you need to ask your doctor for glucagon shots and review it with your family.

My insurance wants me to change from Apidra, Novolog to Humalog. What can I do?

These three rapid-acting (fast-acting) insulins have slight differences, but for practical purposes, we will consider them the same. You can do one unit to one unit conversion. My patients reported that Apidra works slightly faster and lasts a little shorter time. Novolog has a slightly more sugar lowering effect. You will be fine if you start with one to one unit conversion, and then adjust after you've stabilized.

Now we have Fiasp which works even faster. We also consider one to one unit conversion between Fiasp and other analog.

My insurance does not pay for analog (Apidra, Novolog, Humalog) anymore. What can I do?

These days, patients are being squeezed, doctors as well. We are spending more and more time arguing with insurance companies, and most of the time, we still fail. I have to prescribe more and more for Novolin R or Humulin R.

You need to give Novolin R and Humulin R at least 20-30 minutes before you eat since Novolin R and Humulin R start to work slower than analogs.

What is Novolog?

Novolog is a human insulin analog-aspart produced in yeast made by Novo Nordisk. It is usually used for pre-meal insulin, sliding scale (correction), and emergency use. It can be used in type 1, type 2, and gestational diabetes.

What are the dosage forms?

Each presentation contains 100 Units of insulin aspart per mL (U-100)

--10 mL vials

--3 mL PenFill® cartridges 3 mL

-- NOVOLOG® FlexPen® 3 mL

--NOVOLOG® FlexTouch® 3ml (not in all markets)

What is the difference between Novolog and Humalog?

- ➢ Chemically they are different but not too much, compared to native human insulin,
- ➢ Humalog is made in bacteria by Eli Lily; while Novolog is made in yeast by Novo Nordisk.
- ➢ Humalog is recommended to be given 15 minutes before meals, while Novolog is recommended to given 5-10 minutes before meals.
- ➢ Humalog has U-200 (two times more concentrated) while Novolog only has U-100. Humalog U-200 only comes as a pen. Never take insulin from a pen for any other use.
- ➢ My patients reported that Novolog is slightly stronger than Humalog even if using the same units.
- ➢ For most type two diabetes patients, there is no big difference experienced. For type 1 diabetes, a few more patients reported differences.

My insurance switched me from Humalog to Novolog. What should I do?

It is very common these days for insurance companies to demand patients switch from one type of insulin to another. I have patients whose insurance does not even cover insulin analogs (Humalog, Novolog, Apidra) at all. Luckily, for most patients, they do not have major issues when they switch. I do have some patients who have difficulties with unstable sugar. In this case, we would file a petition on the patient's behalf. Sometimes, we are able to help. But sometimes, the insurance will increase the copay so high that patients cannot use it.

From my experience, more patients have issues switching from Novolog to Humalog instead of switching from Humalog to Novolog. Be aware. My patients reported that Novolog works faster and stronger. If you have type 1 diabetes or are very sensitive to insulin, you might want to reduce your dose by 5-10% at the beginning of the switch.

What are the storage instructions for Novolog?
- ➢ Unused vial or pen: refrigerate until expiration date. If frozen, you need to discard it.
- ➢ In-use vial or pen: store in a cool place free of sunlight under 86F (30C) for up to 28 days. Certainly if the expiration date has been reached. it needs to be discarded.
- ➢ Unused pens and vials: if stored at room temperature (below 86F) they need to be discarded after 28 days.

What are the ingredients in Novolog?
Active Ingredient: insulin aspart. Inactive Ingredients: glycerin, phenol, metacresol, zinc, disodium hydrogen phosphate dihydrate, sodium chloride and water for injection.

What is Apidra?
Apidra is a fast-acting insulin analog-glulisine produced in bacteria. In comparison to human insulin, two amino acids are changed. The asparagine at B3 is replaced by lysine; and the lysine at position B27 is replaced by glutamic acid.

What are the dose forms for Apidra?

Apidra 100 units/mL (U-100) is available in 10 mL vials

Apidra SoloStar (prefilled) 3ml

How fast and how long does Apidra work after being subcutaneously injected?

Apidra is a fast-acting insulin. In most patients, it starts to work after ~15 minutes, and has its peak effect at 40-90 mins, and can last three to four hours. Its effect on different patients can vary drastically. Even in the same patient it can be different moment to moment.

What else is in Apidra?

The active ingredient is insulin analog-glulisine.

The inactive ingredients are: tromethamine, metacresol, zinc, polysorbate 20, sodium chloride and water for injection.

My insurance wants me to change from Humalog or Novolog to Apidra. What can I do?

These three fasting insulins have slight differences, but for practical purposes, we will consider them the same. You can do one unit to one unit conversions. My patients reported that Apidra works slightly faster and lasts a little shorter time duration. Novolog has a slightly stronger sugar lowering effect. You will be fine if you start with one unit to one unit conversions, and then adjust after you've stabilized.

What is Fiasp?

Novolog is a human insulin analog-aspart produced in yeast made by Novo Nordisk. It is formulated with niacinamide so that it is being absorbed faster than Novolog alone. It is usually used for pre-meal insulin, sliding scale (correction), and emergency use. It can be used in type 1, type 2.

It is recently approved by FDA. In clinic, at the moment of publishing this book, we have not prescribed it yet. I actually participated in the clinical trial.

What is the clinical advantage of Fiasp?

Fiasp can be given at the beginning of a meal and within 20 minutes of starting your meal for meal insulin coverage. Fiasp is really good for the following situations:

❖ You do not know how much you are going to eat.
❖ You eat at restaurant. You usually do not know when you will be served and how much you will be served.
❖ You forget your pre-meal insulin often until you finish your meal and remember it.

What else in Fiasp?

Fiasp is an aqueous, sterile, clear and colorless solution that contains insulin aspart 100 units/mL, glycerol, phenol, metacresol, zinc, disodium phosphate dihydrate, arginine hydrochloride, niacinamide (vitamin B$_3$), and water for injections.

Fiasp has a pH of 7.1. Hydrochloric acid and/or sodium hydroxide may be added to adjust pH.

How fast and how long does Fiasp work after being subcutaneously injected?

Fiasp starts to have measurable effect on sugar 15-20 minutes after subcutaneously injected. The peak effect time is around 90--130 minutes and lasts 5-7 hours. Insulin can be detected as soon as 2.5 minutes and peak concentration at 63 minutes after injection. The various time is determined by different doses and different patients with variable age, kidney function and liver function.

How is Fiasp supplied?

Fiasp is 100 units of insulin aspart per mL (U-100). It is available as a clear and colorless solution in: 10 mL multiple-dose vials, 3 mL single-patient use Fiasp FlexTouch pen.

How is Fiasp stored?

For unused vial and pen, they need to be stored at refrigerator and not near a freezing compartment until expiration date.

For unused or currently being used vial or pen, if stored at room temperature, they can be used for 28 days.

I am pregnant. Can I continue to use Fiasp?

There is no safety data specifically addressing this issue, but in clinical practice, we use Novolog all the time. Fiasp is Novolog + niacinamide (vitamin B3). If your doctor is comfortable using Novolog during pregnancy, he or she should feel comfortable to using Fiasp.

My doctor change me to Humalog, Novolog, Apidra to Fiasp. What should I do?

As we stated previously, using Fiasp is more convenient. You can use it within 20 minutes after starting your meal for the meal.

For now, we consider 1 unit to 1 unit conversion. However, we do not have enough experience yet. If you prone to have low sugar, I recommend you reduce your dose by 20% and then adjust it as needed.

I am allergic to Fiasp. What can I do?

If you have allergic reaction to Fiasp, you should not use Novolog. If you have reaction to Novolog, you should not use Fiasp. They are basically the same.

You might be able to try Humalog, Apidra or regular insulin. Otherwise, you need to have desensitization. Fortunately this is very rare situation, and I have never met such a patient.

Chapter 11. Regular insulin (Novolin R and Humulin R)

What is the difference between insulin R and analogs (Humalog, Novolog, Apidra, Fiasp)?

Regular Insulin R has the exact same amino acid sequences as your own body produces. When injected subcutaneously, it starts to work after ~30 minutes and peak at three hours, and can last seven hours. Different patients can experience different starting, peak and lasting times. Different injected doses can also have different starting, peak, and lasting times.

Why do we use analogs more than regular R?

When we eat a meal, our body secretes insulin very fast-- within 15 minutes and reaches a peak. Sugar comes down quickly and insulin also comes down quickly. For a balanced meal, insulin will be back to its basal level in around two hours.

As you have seen, the analogs can start to work sooner than R and also come down quicker than R. This matches our eating better, but it is not yet perfect.

Are there any situation where insulin R is preferred?

I prefer to use insulin R in patients with gastroparesis. The matching of absorption and insulin could be better.

I also often use insulin R on type 2 diabetes, especially those with financial difficulties. Insulin R is much more affordable compared to analogs.

I also like to use it on patients with steroid-induced or increased sugar that are temporarily using a high dose steroid.

If administered intravenously in the hospital, I always use insulin R.

Where can I get the lowest price?

You can get 1 vial (1000 units) of Novolin R for a cash price of around $25 from Sam's club or Wal-Mart.

Can I get insulin R in a pen?

No, it only comes in a vial.

My insurance does not pay for analogs (Humalog, Novolog, or Apidra). What can I do?

You can ask your doctor to appeal. The reality is that they make the co-pay so high that you cannot afford it.

Therefore, in most cases, I have to accept it, and the patient has to deal with it. I make sure they:

> ➤ Always check sugar before giving insulin. Checking sugar can prevent low sugar. Not checking is just like driving with your eyes blindfolded. It can be very dangerous especially when taking regular insulin.
> ➤ Try to give it 30 minutes before eating if sugar is not low.
> ➤ If your sugar is already in the range of 70-100 mg/dl, you can consider giving it just before your meal.
> ➤ Always try to eat a meal of low carbs or with complex carbs (Again for type I diabetes, you cannot eat "zero" carb diet).

➢ If dessert cannot missed, I recommend eating it after a meal. Even if you eat fruit as dessert, I recommend you eat it after a meal.
➢ You can start with 1 unit of analog insulin (Humalog, Novolog, Apidra) to insulin R and then titrate afterwards by checking your sugar before your next meal. The dinner insulin dose is adjusted by sugar at bedtime.

Can I mix insulin R with other insulin?

You can mix insulin R with insulin N, and see the instructions in the section on N.

Shunzhong Shawn Bao, MD

Chapter 12. Premix insulin

What are the premix insulins?

The intermediate and short-acting insulins are premixed.
Usually you give them before a meal to control the post meal
sugar and fasting sugar.

What are the regular premix insulins on the market?

Humulin R: Humulin 70/30, The number after Humulin indicates
the percentage of the components, NPH (N) and regular insulin.
N is the insulin mixed with protamine. For details, please see
the section on insulin N. In this premix, 70% is N and 30% is
Humulin R.

Humulin 70/30 comes as a 10 ml vial or 5 pen carton (box) of 3
ml pen. The vial is more affordable.

Humulin R 50/50 has been discontinued by Eli Lily.

Novolin R: Novolin 70/30 also comes as a 10 ml vial or 5 pen
carton (box) of 3 ml pen. The vial is more affordable.

Are there any differences between the Humulin premix and Novolin premix?

We consider them the same.

Novolin 70/30 is more affordable at the Wal-Mart or Sam's club pharmacy. When I am writing this book (2017), a vial of Novolin 70/30 is around $26, and Humulin 70/30 is $145.

What should I know if I am going to use Humulin premix and Novolin premix?

➢ If you have type 1 diabetes, I try my best not to prescribe it, since the risk for low sugar is increased.
➢ If you have a unstable blood sugar, I try my best not to prescribe it.
➢ If your sugar is not low, you need to give Humulin premix or Novolin premix 30 minutes before meal.
➢ You can give two or three times a day before each meal.
➢ You should not miss your meal. If you give the premix before breakfast, the R portion is 30% which controls sugar after breakfast, 70% N peaks at lunch time. If you miss your lunch, you sugar might go low.
➢ Before injection, you need to mix them very well. I ask my patients to roll at least 20 times, but do not shake them. This is very important.

How should I store my regular premix insulin vial?

For vials not in use, store in a refrigerator (36° to 46°F [2° to 8°C]), but not in the freezer until expiration date. Do not use if it has been frozen. If stored at room temperature, below 86°F (30°C) the vial must be discarded after 31 days for Humulin 70/30 and 42 days for Novolin 70/30.

For vials in use, you can store both in a refrigerator or at room temperature for 31 days for Humulin 70/30, 42 days for Novolin 70/30. If stored in a refrigerator, it is recommended that you take it out from the refrigerator to raise it back to room temperature before use.

How should I store my regular premix insulin pen?

For pens not in use, store in a refrigerator (36° to 46°F [2° to 8°C]), but not in the freezer until expiration date. Do not use if it has been frozen. If left at room temperature and below 86°F (30°C) the pen must be discarded after ten days.

For pens in use, store at room temperature, below 86°F (30°C) and the pen must be discarded after ten days, even if the pen still has insulin in it. Again, after you start to use it, do not put it back to refrigerator.

What are the newer versions of premix insulin (analog premix insulin)?

Currently on the market: Humalog Mix 75/25, Humalog Mix 50/50(discontinued), and Novolog Mix 70/30.

Is the newer version mix better than the regular premix insulin?

I think the advantages of using the newer version premix insulin for type 2 diabetes in comparison to the regular version is minimal. The rate of hypoglycemia is reported to be less frequent. However, I never rely on insulin solely to get my patient's sugar back to normal especially for type 2 diabetes.

You can give the newer version a little closer to your meal, since it starts to work slightly faster, 5-20 mins before your meal.

How should the newer premix insulin vial be stored?

For vials not in use: Store in a refrigerator (36° to 46°F [2° to 8°C]), but not in the freezer until expiration date. Do not use if it has been frozen. If stored at room temperature, below 86°F (30°C) the vial must be discarded after 28 days for Humalog Mix 75/25, and 32 days for Novolog 70/30.

For vials in use, you can store both in a refrigerator or room temperature for 28 days (Humalog Mix 75/25, 32 days for Novolog Mix 70/30). If stored in a refrigerator, it is recommended that you take it out from the refrigerator to raise it back to room temperature before use.

How should I store the newer version premix pen?

For pens not in use, store in a refrigerator (36° to 46°F [2° to 8°C]), but not in the freezer until expiration date. Do not use if it has been frozen. If left at room temperature and below 86°F (30°C) the pen must be discarded after ten days for Humalog Mix pen, and 14 days for Novolog Mix pen.

For pens in use, store at room temperature, below 86°F (30°C), and the pen must be discarded after 10 days for Humalog Mix pen, and 14 days for Novolog Mix pen, even if the pen still has insulin in it. Again, after you start to use it, do not put it back in the refrigerator.

Can you give me the summary for all the storage conditions?

All pens and vials not in use need to be stored in a refrigerator at 36° to 46°F until expiration.

	Not in Use or in-use at room temperature	In-use at refrigerator
Humulin Mix Vial	31 days	31 days
Humulin Mix Pen	10 days	Not recommended
Novolin Mix Vial	42 days	42 days
Novolin Mix Pen	10 days	Not recommended
Humalog Mix Vial	28 days	28 days
Humalog Mix Pen	10 days	Not recommended
Novolog Mix Vial	32 days	32 days
Novolog Mix Pen	14 days	Not recommended

I am taking premix two times a day, before breakfast and dinner. I forgot my morning dose. What should I do?

It is very important that you have a scheduled life if you are taking premix insulin. Premix is hard to adjust and catch up. Most time, we have to let you just miss that dose.

One way is to take the morning dose before lunch. Then you might need to reduce pre-dinner dose if you pre-dinner is not high, since the N part works at dinner.

If I missed my pre-dinner dose, what can I do?

If you forget your dinner does, your sugar might go up. Depending on your sugar, give a half or full dose ASAP. Usually, the analog insulin after the meal dose works well. In most cases, you should be okay, but premixes have another peak that will falls 4-8 hours later after you give the injection. If you give your insulin too much later, your sugar might drop around midnight or the early morning. If are you prone to having low sugar, I strongly recommend checking your sugar.

My sugar is high, can I have a sliding scale using premix insulin?

It is not recommended to have a sliding scale (correction scale) using premix insulin. The premix insulin lasts too long and might easily cause low sugar.

Which premix is the most affordable?

Novolin mx 70/30 is the most affordable currently. I cost around $27 at Sam's club or Wal-mart.

Chapter 13. More detailed plans for adjusting insulin dosage

I am using basal insulin and my sugar is 100 mg/dl. Should I give myself insulin or not?

Diabetes is a severe disease and you have to make decisions every day at every moment. As a diabetes patient you have to learn every day. Here I will just provide some general guidance. This is not bulletproof. It is okay to develop your own protocol with your doctor.

Here are a few points to consider.

- ➤ What is your sugar target?
- ➤ What is your response history?
- ➤ What is your current and near future physical activity?
- ➤ What are your diet/snack considerations?
- ➤ Are you on any medications that might increase or decrease your sugar?

What is my sugar target if I am taking basal insulin?

Your sugar target should be determined by your physical condition and your history of hypoglycemia. I mainly consider your risk for hypoglycemia.

Forming an appropriate target is not an easy task. Other important factors to consider are life expectancy, disease duration, presence or absence of micro- and macrovascular complications (retinopathy, nephropathy, history of vascular stents, bypass, heart attack), CVD risk factors (smoking, high cholesterol, family history, etc.), comorbid conditions (liver disease, kidney disease, and heart disease, stroke) and the patient's psychological status, as well as the patient's cognitive status. I also take patient's living status and social support into consideration and his or her personal life status.

If you are taking basal insulin, I am recommend you to check your sugar at least 2 times a day.

For detailed proposed targets, please see the question in Chapter 1. <u>What is a proposed target of sugar and A1c?</u>

I am taking Toujeo, Lantus, Basaglar, or Tresiba as a basal insulin once a day at night, and my night time (bedtime) sugar is in the target, what is your general guideline?

> ➤ First, you need to look at the bedtime sugar. In this case, it is in the target.
> ➤ Consider what you ate for current and previous dinner.
> ➤ Then look at previous two day's morning sugar
> ➤ I usually set the maximum dose at 60-80 units

Life is complicated. Lots of things can happen. You can have thousands of scenarios. I ran a few examples (I cannot list all the scenarios since it is endless) in the following table.

	Night sugar	Previous Morning sugar	Previous Dinner amount	Today's dinner amount	Action
Scenario 1	In target	In target	usual	usual	Same dose
Scenario 2	In target	>target	usual	usual	Increase 2 U every 2-3 days
Scenario 3	In target	>target	larger	usual	Same dose
Scenario 4	In target	<target, but >70	usual	usual	Reduce 2 U every 2-3 days
Scenario 5	In target	<70, but>50	usual	usual	Reduce dose by 50%
Scenario 6	In target	<70, but>50	smaller	usual	Reduce dose by 30%
Scenario 7	In target	<50	usual	usual	Reduce dose by 50%, or hold for type 2

I am taking Toujeo, Lantus, Basaglar, or Tresiba as a basal insulin once a day at night, and my night time (bedtime) sugar is above the target. What is your general guideline?

> First, you need to look at your bedtime sugar. In this case, the bedtime sugar is high.
> Consider what you ate for dinner.
> Then look at previous two day's morning sugar.
> I set the maximum dose as 60-80 units.

Life is complicated. Lots of things can happen. You can have thousands of scenarios. I ran a few examples in the following table.

	Night sugar	Previous Morning sugar	Previous Dinner amount	Today's dinner amount	Action
Scenario 1	> target	In target	usual	usual	Same dose or increase by 10%
Scenario 2	> target	>target	usual	usual	Increase 2 U every 2-3 days
Scenario 3	>target	>target	larger	usual	Increase 2 U every 2-3 days
Scenario 4	>target	<target, but >70	usual	usual	*Reduce 2 U every 2-3 days
Scenario 5	>target	<70, but>50	usual	usual	*Reduce dose by 50%
Scenario 6	>target	<70, but>50	smaller	usual	*Reduce dose by 30%
Scenario 7	> target	<50	usual	usual	*Reduce dose by 50%, or hold for type 2

- For scenarios 4-7, I strongly recommend you discuss with your doctor about changing the regimen. You might need to switch your night time dose to morning, or split the dose.

I am taking Toujeo, Lantus, Basaglar, or Tresiba as a basal insulin once a day at night, and my night time (bedtime) sugar is below the target. What is your general guideline?

> ➤ First, you need to look at your bedtime sugar. In this case, it is below the target. In other words, it is too low.
> ➤ Consider what you ate for dinner.
> ➤ Then look at the previous two day's morning sugar
> ➤ I set the maximum dose as 60-80 units.

Life is complicated. Lots of things can happen. You can have thousands of scenarios. I ran a few examples in the following table.

	Night sugar	Previous Morning sugar	Previous Dinner amount	Today's dinner amount	Action
Scenario 1	< target, but>110	In target	usual	usual	*Same dose or reduce by 20%
Scenario 2	< target, but>110	>target	usual	usual	*Keep the same
Scenario 3	<target, but>110	>target	larger	usual	*keep the same
Scenario 4	<target, but>110	<target, but >70	usual	usual	*Reduce 30%
Scenario 5	<target, but>110	<70, but>50	usual	usual	*Reduce dose by 50%
Scenario 6	<target, but>110	<70, but>50	smaller	usual	*Reduce dose by 50%
Scenario 7	< target	<50	usual	usual	*Reduce dose by 80%, or hold for type 2

*For these scenarios, I also recommend the following:

- For night time sugar <110, I recommend small snacks (15 g of carbs).

- For less than target but>110, you have an option to eat a small snack if you're prone to having low sugar.
- Discuss with your physician to get more individualized plan of action. See Chapter 1 for more information.

I am taking pre-meal insulin, my morning sugar is too high. What can I do?

➢ Make sure to see if there's anything you can do to make it better tomorrow.
  ○ Eat a smaller portion of a dinner
  ○ Eat a little early
  ○ Go for a walk instead of sitting down watching TV or going to bed after dinner
  ○ Check midnight and 2:00 am sugar to make sure it is not low
➢ You might need to increase your basal insulin by 2 units every 2-3 days as we discussed above. If you are taking too much basal insulin already, you might consider increase your premeal insulin before dinner.
➢ If you are taking your basal insulin in the morning, then you might want to move your basal insulin to be given at night.
➢ If you are taking your basal insulin in the morning, then you can also consider to split your basal doses, morning and night dose.
➢ You might want to eat less that morning.
➢ You can also give yourself a correction dose.

My pre-lunch sugar is too high. What can I do?

➢ Try to make better diet choices tomorrow
  ○ Eat a smaller portion of breakfast.
  ○ Do not eat something both high in fat and high in carbs like pizza or combination of high fat and high carbs.
  ○ Do not eat a snack especially too close to lunch.
  ○ Do some activity in-between breakfast and lunch.

➢ You might need additional fast-acting insulin as correction dose (sliding scale).
➢ You might want to eat less for lunch.
➢ You might want to have more afternoon physical activity.
➢ If your pre-lunch sugar is persistently high, you might want to increase your tomorrow's pre-breakfast insulin by 2 units every one to two days.

My pre-dinner sugar is too high. What can I do?

➢ Make sure to see if there's anything you can do better for tomorrow
  ○ Do not eat too large a lunch tomorrow
  ○ Do not eat something both high in fat and high in carbs-like pizza
  ○ Do not eat a snack especially too close to dinner
➢ Do more physical activity.
➢ You might want to add a correction dose (sliding scale) before dinner.
➢ If your pre-dinner sugar is persistently high, you might need to increase your pre-lunch fast-acting insulin by 2 units every one to two days.
➢ You might want to eat less for dinner.
➢ You might want to have more physical activity after dinner.

My morning sugar is too low. What can I do?

➢ You might want to reduce basal insulin, if there is a pattern (see above).
➢ You might consider reducing your pre-dinner insulin by 2 or more units, if there is a pattern.
➢ For today, you can reduce your pre-breakfast insulin dose (more details below).
➢ For today, you might want to give insulin after the meal.

My pre-lunch sugar is too low. What can I do?

➤ You might want to reduce tomorrow's pre-breakfast insulin if there is a pattern.
➤ For today, you can reduce your pre-lunch insulin dose (more details below).
➤ For today, you might want to give insulin after the meal.

My pre-dinner sugar is too low. What can I do?

➤ You might want to reduce tomorrow's pre-lunch insulin if there is a pattern.
➤ For today, you can reduce your pre-dinner insulin dose (more details below).
➤ For today, you might want to give insulin after the meal.
➤ Certainly you always want to check your bedtime sugar.

What are your general recommendations for low pre-meal sugar on that day?

➤ You need to have a target, so you know if your sugar is too high, too low or acceptable. For details about target, please refer to Chapter 1.

Sugar level (mg/dl)	What to do?
< target, but higher than 70	Take your usual dose and eat your meal right away
<70, >50	Eat your meal, and consider taking half a dose after your meal
<50	You can treat your low sugar or eat your meal without giving any insulin

What are your general recommendations for daily adjustment of pre-meal insulin?

➤ The dose can be adjusted based on what you are eating and how much you are eating. Usually the more carbs you are eating, the more insulin you should give.

➤ If you are not eating, do not give any pre-meal insulin. Sliding scale (correction dose) can be given if your sugar is high.

➤ When you don't know how much you are going to eat, you might give a small portion before your meal and give the rest immediately after you eat. Fiasp is licensed to be given within 20 minutes after starting a meal.

➤ When you are unsure, it is always better to give less insulin than to give too much.

➤ If you are eating out, always wait to give your pre-meal insulin until after you see the food. You never know when or how much you will be served. Also always track what you ate and add more insulin as needed.

➤ Consider the physical activity taken before and after your meal. Mostly you need to consider your after meal physical activity. If your physical activity is higher than usual you can consider reducing your pre-meal insulin. Pre-meal activity also affects your post meal sugar but much less. If you have prolonged or an unusual level of physical activity before the meal, you can also consider reducing the meal insulin dose.

➤ If you have pain or severe stress, most likely you need to increase your pre-meal insulin. Here comes the art rather than science part. You can consider increasing your pre-meal insulin by 20% to try it out. Certainly, you need to closely monitor your sugar. Ideally I recommend you wear a CGM (continuous glucose monitor).

Chapter 14. Insulin use for shift-workers

Why does shift work pose an extra challenge in using insulin?

Ideally, diabetes patients especially if on insulin, need to live a scheduled daily life. A shift worker's constantly changing life poses a special challenge. Your diurnal rhythm, insulin sensitivity, physical activity and your pattern of eating all change. Your sugar tends to go high or low much more easily.

What can I do to make my insulin use safer and more effective as a shift worker?

- ➢ Although your shift may constantly change, try to find a certain pattern, or make a pattern, and try to keep it stable.
- ➢ Tell your treating doctor what your working time, sleeping time, and eating time are, and specifically what you do during and off the shift and on off days.
- ➢ Your treating physician can help you to make a plan. Plans are very important so that you can be prepared.
- ➢ You might need to have different plans for on shift, off shift, and off days.
- ➢ Tell your colleagues about your diabetes and your insulin treatment and educate them on how to help you if your sugar is too low and/or you become mentally impaired.

The reason you want to tell your colleagues is that usually night shifts have fewer people working, and if you tell them, they might be able to pay more attention to you.

➢ Always be prepared to have something for low sugar since the night shift might have less resources available to you.

➢ I also recommend you to have a CGM (continuous glucose monitor) which can check your sugar every five minutes 24 hours a day, seven days a week. You can "see" your sugar number trending up or down. It can also give you a warning.

➢ I also recommend an insulin pump if possible, an insulin pump can be set to give different basal rate, insulin carb ratio, sensitivity at different time.

I am a shift worker with type 2 diabetes, and my doctor said I need to be on insulin. What is your recommendation?

I have a few ways to deal with it depending on your preference, response, and resources (insurance) to pay. There are different shift types, but the most common are 8-hour and 12-hour shifts.

➢ If your insurance pays for Tresiba, I would try it first. Since Tresiba allows you to take a catch up dose up to 12 hours late. If those days that you are working and not able to take your dose, if you use Tresiba, you can always take a catch-up dose.

➢ If your insurance doesn't pay for Tresiba and if your insurance pays any other long-acting like Lantus, Toujeo, you can try to give your insulin at the same time. A difficulty will arise if you have a rotating shift. Then it is not ideal to wait to give yourself shot.

➢ If you have a rotating shift, I have the following options for you:
   ○ Option 1: you can use any of the basal insulins- NPH, Levemir, Lantus, Basaglar. Give either of them three times a day at the same time instead of

once a day. For those rotating shifts, you should rotate every 8 hours.
- Option 2: if your shift rotates every 12 hours, then you can give your shot every day once a day or every 12 hours. This kind of rotating shift usually does not create too many problem if you are on top of it.
- Option 3: if your insurance pays for an insulin pump, this can be a good option for you. Just set up your insulin pump to deliver your different basal insulin at different shifts.
- Option 4: If your insurance covers V-go, (a device that delivers daily basal and bolus insulin), it may be able to deliver insulin like an insulin pump, although it is not one. You have to change it daily however.
- Option 5: Instead of giving a basal regime, you can try giving bolus before you eat. This way, when you are awake and eating, you give yourself insulin. There are lots of ways to give. You can give any fast-acting insulin, like regular insulin, Apidra, Humalog, Novolog or Fiasp. If you feel giving insulin at work is not convenient, you can try to give it as an inhaled insulin -Afrezza.

I have type 1 diabetes and I am a shift worker. What is my best option?

If you have type 1 diabetes, I strongly recommend getting an insulin pump. This is truly the best option for you. You usually can program it in such a way that gives you different basal rate, different insulin carb rate and different sensitivity on different shifts and on off days to match your basal and bolus requirement better.

Now we have a semi closed-loop insulin pump (artificial pancreas) which might even do a better job. If you cannot get a closed-loop insulin pump, try your best to get the CGM (continuous glucose monitor).

Shunzhong Shawn Bao, MD

If you really do not like to have a pump, I would like to recommend V-go for you. Again, this is a device capable of delivering both basal and bolus for you. Remember, you have to change this V-go every day.

If giving shots is not convenient to you, you can also try inhaled insulin for your bolus needs.

I have type 1 diabetes and I am a shift worker and have to stay on shots. What is your recommendation?

For bolus (pre-meal insulin), you should have no problem. When you eat, you can check your sugar and give yourself bolus. You need to pay attention to the days you are on and off days. You might need a different amount of insulin for the same carb you eat (different insulin carb ratio). Again, if possible, ask your doctor for a CGM (continuous glucose monitor).

For basals (basal insulins), I would recommend the following options for you.

> ➢ Option 1: if your insurance will pay for Tresiba, I would recommend this for you since you do not have to give yourself insulin at exact time every day. You have a 12 hours window to give. For details, please discuss this with your physician.
> ➢ Option 2, if you are awake every 12 or every 24 hours, then you can either give yourself basal every 12 hours or every 24 hours.
> ➢ If your sleep time is chaotic, then I strongly recommend starting an insulin pump. You can also use V-go to deliver your insulin. If you developed type 1 diabetes in childhood, you need to be on both pre-meal bolus insulin in addition to basal insulin. However, if you developed type 1 diabetes in adulthood, then you might be able to try only using bolus insulin if you have residual beta cell function.

Chapter 15. Truck Drivers and Insulin

Can I be a truck driver or continue to be a truck driver if I have Type 2 diabetes and use insulin?

Maybe, but you have to "jump through some hoops" for this to occur. You will have to apply for the Federal Diabetes Exemption through the FMCSA. See below under, "Obtaining an FMCSA Diabetes Waiver".

What is FMCSA Diabetes Waiver?

If you want to be a commercial drive r or continue to be a commercial driver while on insulin, you need to apply for FMCSA (Federal Motor Carrier Safety Agency) diabetes waiver. The Federal Diabetes and Vision Exemption Programs have specific requirements, as well as requests for hearing and seizure exemptions. These requests may include medical exams, employment history, driving experience, and motor vehicle records which must be submitted with the application. The Agency will make a final decision within 180 days of receipt of the complete application.

For more information, please visit:

https://www.fmcsa.dot.gov/medical/driver-medical-requirements/driver-exemption-programs

From a medical point of view, how do I prepare for the exemption application?

1. You need to bring a Certifying Medical Examiner Evaluation letter to the appointment with the medical

examiner for him/her to review prior to performing the examination. Additionally, the applicant must bring a copy of his/her 5-year medical history to the examination for the medical examiner to review. You can find a certified examiner here: https://nationalregistry.fmcsa.dot.gov/NRPublicUI/Drivers.seam

2. You need to go to your endocrinologist to obtain records and forms.
3. You need to go to your ophthalmologist to obtain records and forms.

If you do not see your doctor as scheduled and regularly, these can be daunting tasks.

If you need information about this, you can visit: https://dotmedicalexaminerblog.com/2014/03/14/how-to-apply-to-the-federal-diabetes-exemption-program/

How will endocrinologists evaluate to assess your diabetes control?

If you have one of the following, you might not be able to pass the endocrinologist's evaluation.

The form for endocrinologists is long, but most importantly, you cannot have the following conditions:

- The person with diabetes must not have had one or more hypoglycemic episodes in the past 12 months, or two or more occurrences in the past five years resulting in:
  1. Seizure
  2. Loss of Consciousness
  3. Need for assistance from another person
  4. Period of Confusion
- The person with diabetes must not have signs of end (severe) organ damage including:

1. Retinopathy
2. Macular Degeneration
3. Peripheral Neuropathy--most patients have it. So how to quantify this depends on your endocrinologist's judgement.
4. Congestive Heart Disease
5. Stroke
6. Peripheral Vascular Disease
7. Kidney Failure

Again, you need your endocrinologist to evaluate your risk for hypoglycemia, your sugar's stability, your compliance to regimens, and of any peripheral neuropathy.

What can I do if my endocrinologist is not willing to fill out the form?

They may be refusing for one of the following reasons:

1. If you have really uncontrolled or unstable sugar, with high A1c
2. If you have had severe hypoglycemia once in the past 12 months or two times in the past five years.
3. If you have severe peripheral neuropathy
4. Or he or she has not been following your regimen closely.

If you do not think you have any of above situations, you might want to ask for your medical records and find another endocrinologist to fill the form for you.

I saw a patient two years ago who then failed to follow up. One day he came back with the form for me to fill out. I did not complete the form since I did not have enough information. Two weeks later, I saw him again in the hospital. He drove into the opposite lane and killed a lady. He survived. This is very important. Life or death consequences.

What else can I do if I cannot get my endocrinologist on board?

Here are my recommendations:

1. Start to take care of yourself very seriously, check sugar, follow my low carb, low meat, low calorie diet, and do as many activities as you can.
2. Check your sugar as needed and maintain a good record, so you can show it to your endocrinologist.
3. If possible, get a CGM (continuous glucose monitoring) which can really help you stay out of trouble.
4. Discuss the possibility of using different medications like non-insulin injections (GLP-1 agonists), if appropriate.
5. You can also ask for other oral medications like SGLT2 antagonists, for example, Farxiga, Jardiance, Invokana and their combinations if appropriate.
6. Note: suggestions 4.and 5., only pertain to type 2 diabetes.

I have type 2 diabetes, and I am a truck driver. What can I do as a truck driver to avoid insulin in the future?

It is not easy to be a truck driver and take care of your diabetes. You have to sit long hours with lack of activity. You do not have good choices in terms of eating.

However, you can still make a few changes. Here are a few recommendations:

1. Get a cooler to bring your own food instead of eating fast food at truck stops.

2. Every few hours, get out of the truck and run for 15 minutes or just walking. Studies show that if you are healthy enough, a few minutes of burst exercises at the

maximal intensity equals moderate intensity exercise at a longer time.

3. If possible, you can also put exercise equipment in the back of your truck, so you can do your exercises at the truck stop.

4. You might want to ask your fellow drivers to see what they do to exercise.

5. You can visit some websites for some ideas, such as http://www.livestrong.com/article/462361-exercises-that-truckers-can-do-in-their-vehicle/; http://truckersfund.org/5-ways-exercise-truck/; and youtube videos: https://www.youtube.com/watch?v=mKMC63ysO9w.

6. Check your sugars and keep up with all your doctor appointments.

7. If possible, get a CGM (continuous glucose monitor). When you can see your sugar going up, you hopefully will change your behavior.

8. Do not smoke which in diabetic patients greatly increases the risk of cardiovascular disease.

9. Make sure your blood pressure is well controlled.

10. If your doctor agrees, you should take aspirin daily.

Chapter 16. Questions about high and low blood sugar levels and dealing with steroids

What symptoms or signs might indicate low sugar?

When sugar is low, your adrenaline is secreted. This causes you to have palpitations, perspiration (sweat), pale skin, shakiness, tingling, anxiety, irritability, slurred speech and hunger.

You might wake up drenched in perspiration and/or crying out during sleep.

As hypoglycemia worsens, you might develop confusion, abnormal behavior or both. You may also experience the inability to concentrate, and difficulty in completing routine tasks. Visual disturbances may occur such as blurred vision. If these are severe enough, they can cause seizures, loss of consciousness, or even death.

What should I do if I feel my sugar is low?

You should stop whatever you are doing especially if you are driving. You also need to check your sugar and treat yourself.

Shunzhong Shawn Bao, MD

How should I treat low sugar?

Usually, it is recommended to have 15 grams of carbs and then wait for 15 minutes to make sure your sugar is back to normal.

Here are some examples of 15 grams of carbs:

· Three glucose tablets

· One-half cup (4 ounces or 118 ml) of fruit juice

· Four ounces of regular, non-diet soda

· Five hard candies

· One tablespoon (tbsp.) or 15 ml of sugar - plain or

dissolved in water

· One tbsp. (15 ml) of honey

If your sugar is not back up over 70 after 15-20 minutes, you need to repeat the process.

I recommend that you always have some glucose tablets in your purse or in your car's glove compartment.

Depending on the situation, there are lots of other ways to treat your low sugar. If your sugar is low just before your meal, you can just go ahead and have your meal. Depending on your sugar level, and diabetes regimen, you need to adjust your medications.

When you see your doctor, you need to report this situation.

What should I do if my sugar is low and I do not feel it?

Here, we assume that you do not have any hypoglycemic signs or symptoms, but your meter shows that you have sugar below 60-70. Here are two scenarios.

Scenario 1: Your sugar is not actually low, but your sugar meter is showing that it is low. In other words, the meter you are using may not be accurate. Occasionally, glucometers can have problems with accuracy.

Based on new FDA regulations, if a patient's blood sugar is below 75, the reading should be within plus or minus 15 of the actual sugar, 95% of the time. For example, if your actual blood sugar is at 70, the meter is acceptable within the new FDA guidelines to show 60.

In these situations, you need to make a judgment call. If your sugar is below 60, but close to 60, and if you are feeling fine, and if you are going to eat, you can continue your current regimen.

If you are on a multiple daily insulin shot regimen, you can give half of your pre-meal insulin before the meal and give the other half of your insulin when you eat or after you eat.

Scenario 2: If you have hypoglycemia unawareness, then you need to be more cautious. You have to treat every low sugar reading as an actual low sugar condition.

What should I do if I cannot feel when my sugar is low?

This is called hypoglycemia unawareness, which is very serious and has severe consequences.

Here are the five recommendations I usually give to my patients who have hypoglycemia unawareness:

1. Ask for CGM (continuous glucose monitoring) if your insurance will pay and/or you can afford it. This device can be a lifesaver for patients with hypoglycemia unawareness.
2. Check your sugar more often, especially before you drive (ideally not drive); check your sugar before and after exercise in addition to before meals and at bedtime.
3. Use an insulin pump that will shut down if your sugar is low.
4. Talk to your doctor and he or she will raise your sugar levels, and in most cases, your sense of hypoglycemia will return.
5. Create a higher diabetes control target.

When should I use the glucagon shot my doctor prescribed for me?

This is not for you to use. This is for family members or other bystanders to use to treat your low sugar if you become unconscious and are unable to eat or drink. Do not use it if your sugar is simply low.

How should I use the glucagon shot?

Educate your family or whoever may be able to help you in emergency situations. Here are three recommendations:

1. After you fill the prescription, open it to review with your family or the people who might be available to help you.
2. Watch a YouTube instructional video together about how to use it and when to use it.
3. If one of your kits has expired, do not throw it away. You can use this kit to practice. Do not inject yourself; inject into a sponge or something safe.

Here are two things to remember about glucagon shots.

1. The injection sites are the same sites as insulin injection sites, like abdomen, outer shoulder, and outer thigh.

2. Turn the patient to his or her left or right side since glucagon may cause vomiting.

If you have an episode of unconsciousness and you used your glucagon shot, you need to go to the ER to be evaluated. They will make sure your sugar is stable and get it back up if necessary. After this, you need to visit your doctor's office to see if your regimen needs to be adjusted.

When should I go to the hospital if I have low sugar?

If you have prolonged or severe episodes of hypoglycemia, such as

- ➢ Having treated it three times (with 15 g of carbs) and you have been unable to get it back up, you relapse into low sugar sometime in the same day.
- ➢ If your low sugar is so severe that you lose consciousness or you have a seizure.
- ➢ Or for whatever reason. It is okay to be fully checked.
- ➢ If you used your glucagon (see above when and how to use it), then you should go.

What should I do to prevent hypoglycemia?

- ➢ Know what kind of insulin you are taking, long-acting, short-acting, or intermediate insulin, when it will start to work, how long it will work.
- ➢ Do not miss an insulin dose. When you miss a dose, your sugar will be high, and then your doctor will increase your dose and the chance of developing low sugar will increase.
- ➢ Do not miss your meals.
- ➢ Be careful when new medications are added. Some medication might increase your insulin secretion, or action, or temper your body's response to low sugar.

➤ Anticipate your near future activity. If you are giving your basal insulin in the morning, and you are going to do lots physical work today, you can try reducing your insulin dose by 30%. If you are giving your basal insulin the night before, you might give the same dose, but eat a little more during the day. If your activity is very strenuous, then you might need to reduce your bedtime long-acting also beside you eat more during the day.

➤ Always have a plan, especially if you are taking insulin, like when to reduce your dose, when to hold (see previous chapters for details).

➤ If your insurance pays for it, you should get a CGM (continuous glucose monitor). My patients really like it.

➤ Immediately check your sugar if you think your sugar is dropping.

What medications might increase my chance of having low sugar?

All antidiabetic agents, if in combination with insulin, will increase the risk for low sugar. Other drugs like salicylates (increase endogenous insulin secretion), sulfonamide antibiotics, monoamine oxidase inhibitors, fluoxetine, disopyramide, fibrates, propoxyphene, pentoxifylline, ACE inhibitors, angiotensin II receptor blocking agents, and somatostatin analogs (e.g., octreotide) might cause low sugar or your sense of low sugar.

My morning sugar is always high. What can I do?

This is really frequently asked question. I answered this question in other sections. I want to repeat myself here.

There are a few reasons you might have high morning sugar.

The most common reasons are that you might have eaten too much at dinner or that you might have eaten too late at night. If this is the case, certainly, I recommend that you cut down your night meal portions and move your dinnertime earlier. Ideally, it would be good if you can take a walk after your dinner.

The second most common reason is that you ate a bedtime snack. It is not a good idea to have a bedtime snack if your sugar is not low. I do not know who first started this idea. Bedtime snacks are the cause for weight gain. Certainly, if your sugar is low, you need to have a snack; otherwise, you do not need to eat. If your sugar consistently goes low during the night or morning, your regimen needs to be adjusted.

The third reason could be caused by the "dawn effect". This is more common in teenagers. In the morning, hormones like cortisol and growth hormones are secreted to prepare you for the morning, and these hormones increase your sugar. If this is the case, your doctor will adjust your regimen accordingly.

The fourth reason is that your long-acting insulin may not be long enough or the dose is too low. You might need to discuss this with your treating doctor to see if a change in your insulin regimen is necessary. Your doctor may increase your night time insulin, or change it to a different long-acting insulin, or change it to twice daily, especially if you are taking Levemir.

The last and most important cause, is the Somogyi effect. This effect happens when low sugar is followed by a rebound of high sugar. If your night sugar goes low, your body will secrete stress hormones like cortisol, growth hormone, and adrenaline to raise your blood sugar. It can overshoot and cause your blood sugar to be high. This is actually not so common in my experience, but it is important to recognize it when it happens.

As you can see, if your sugar is too low already, and if your insulin increases, your sugar will go even lower. However, if you do not have hypoglycemia unawareness, if your sugar is too low, you will wake up sweating, with tremors, clammy, and a rapid heartbeat. If the Somogyi effect is suspected, I usually ask my patients to check their sugar at bedtime, midnight, 2 a.m., 4 a.m., and 6-8 a.m. If midnight or early morning low sugar is confirmed, then you are said to have the "Somogyi effect." You need to discuss this with your doctor and have your regimen adjusted.

When do I need to check urine ketones?

Ketones are produced when your body does not have enough insulin to use glucose as fuel, so it instead uses your fat as fuel. If severe enough, it can cause ketoacidosis which can be life threatening.

Ketoacidosis usually occurs in type 1 diabetes patients, although it can sometimes occur in type 2 diabetes patients.

However, in the clinic, we usually do not discuss ketones if you have type 2 diabetes and have never had ketoacidosis before.

Under the following conditions, or any time you think you might have ketoacidosis, please check your urine ketones. You can buy test strips from your local pharmacy without a prescription, although you can also ask your doctor for a prescription. These are the symptoms:

- You feel sick, especially with nausea, vomiting, or abdominal pain.
- You cannot get your sugar under control, if you have type 1 diabetes and your sugar is persistently higher than 250.
- If you have fever, >100° F
- If your skin is flushed
- If your breath smells "fruity"
- If you feel like your thinking is "foggy"
- If you are taking those SGLT2 inhibitors like Invokana, Jardiance, Farxiga, and if you have any of above

What do I need to do if my ketones are positive?
You need to call your doctor.

Most likely, you will need to go to the ER to make sure you are properly treated, especially if your sugar cannot be controlled. You may have severe dehydration.

What should I do if I have nausea and vomiting and I am unable to keep anything down?
Many reasons can cause nausea and vomiting. If this is the first time in a long time, you need to go to the emergency room or call your doctor immediately, because you may be developing ketoacidosis. This is when you need to check your urine ketones.

If you have recurrent nausea and vomiting, you may have gastroparesis.

What should I do if my sugar goes above 500 after a steroid shot?
Steroids are commonly used for many conditions, and they can increase your sugar significantly. It is not uncommon for your sugar to go over 500 after a steroid shot.

Here are the things you can do:

First, you need to make sure you do not have any other illnesses, such as a cough or a urinary problem. If you feel really bad, go to the ER.

Otherwise, you can try the following:

- Call your doctor or visit your doctor's office for advice.

- Drink plenty of water.
- Cut down on all carbs you are eating.
- Eat only green vegetables.
- If you are taking insulin already, increase your pre-meal insulin by 20-30% at first and then double your dose, and then continue sliding scale (corrections).
- If you are taking basal insulins like Lantus, Basaglar, Toujeo or Tresiba, you can also try to take 30% more. However, if you are taking them at night, you need to move to the morning or add one dose in the morning to prevent overnight low sugar.
- If you are taking Levemir, you might be able to take more. Every day you can try to increase by 10%, up to 100% and give it in the morning.
- If you are taking NPH (N) or premix, you can increase the morning dose up to 100%
- If you cannot get it down, go to the ER or your doctor's office.
- You need to check sugar often and get advice from your doctor's office.

I am on steroids. Do you have some general recommendations?

➢ This certainly depends on how much steroids you are on, for what reason you are on steroids, and what and how much you eat.
➢ If possible, you need to reduce your carbs to a minimum (If you have type I diabetes, you cannot eat "zero carb" diet.
➢ Drink lots of water.
➢ Increase physical activity if possible.
➢ You can consider increasing your pre-meal insulin by 20%. If it is still high, you can try up to 50% or double it. Your response is affected by many factors, such as the amount of steroids you are taking and how many carbs you are eating, etc.
➢ Depending on what kind of steroid and through which route it is given, it might take days to wean the effect of steroids.

➤ I also recommend other medications like GLP-1 agonists such as Victoza, Trulicity or Bydureon to reduce your appetite if appropriate.

➤ I also recommend other medications like SGLT2 antagonists like Jardiance, Invokana and Farxiga if appropriate.

➤ I also recommend other medications like Acarbose to reduce your carb absorption.

➤ Steroids also increase your appetite. Sometimes, I also recommend appetite suppressants.

➤ You are advised to consult your diabetes doctor before starting steroids.

What should I do if my sugar goes over 500 and I am not taking steroids?

Do not panic. Calm down and ask yourself if there was anything you ate or did that may have caused the sugar spike. Try to identify the cause and see if the cause can be corrected. If you are fine and your sugar is high, you can try to correct the cause and use the sliding scale to see if you can get the sugar down.

If you are only on basal insulin, you can try to give 30% of basal insulin in the morning.

If you have sugar over 500, and you have a fever, chest pain, nausea and vomiting, or severe weakness or even confusion, you need to go to the ER.

Whatever you do, you need to let your doctor know and they might have different advice for you.

What are the common reasons for sugar to go over 500?

Based on my patients' reports, the following 10 reasons are common:

1. Steroid use.
2. Common colds, with cold medications. Some antibiotics can cause sugar spikes.
3. Forgetting to take insulin.
4. Eating or drinking something really sweet. Something with lots of carbs even if it claims to have "no sugar."
5. Some kind of infection, such as UTI (urinary tract infection).
6. Alcohol- worse if alcohol is mixed with sugar.
7. Insulin pump problems (insertion cannula kinked, or inserted into a scar).
8. Expired insulin.
9. Dehydration.
10. Stress/pain.

I am on an insulin pump. My sugar goes over 500. What should I do?

As we discussed above, you can have any of the ten possibilities or in combination. You need to think back to see what might have happened or is happening. Here are some points related more to patients on an insulin pump.

➢ Most likely you have type 1 diabetes or have severe insulin deficiency. You need premeal insulin. When you eat anything with carbs, you need to give some insulin if eating is not for treating low sugar. I have patients whose sugar go to over 500 just eating a small cookie or drinking small cup of fruit juice.

➢ If you are feeling fine, you can try to give bolus based on sensitivity. If your meter shows Hi (too high to measure), you can try to give 50% more insulin based on the sensitivity. Check your sugar after 20-30 minutes, if your sugar is not coming down, you need to change your infusion set. I recommend that you change your insulin also, since it might be degraded. I would start a new bottle.

➢ If your sugar is not coming down after you changed your insulin and the infusion set, you need to give yourself insulin shot subcutaneously based on your sensitivity. Therefore, even if you are on insulin pump, you always need to purchase some insulin syringes for occasions like this.

➤ Certainly if you are not feeling well and especially if you are not able to get your sugar down, you need to go to the ER to make sure you are not developing DKA.
➤ Whatever you do, you need to closely monitor your sugar until stabilized. It is not uncommon to overcorrect and cause low sugar.

What should I do if for no reason my sugar goes over 500?

You need to call your doctor immediately or go to the ER.

Diabetics can have silent heart attacks which can cause your sugar to go over 500.

What should I do if my sugar is persistently higher than 250 and I do not feel well?

If you have ketone strips, check your ketones to see if you are developing DKA (diabetic ketoacidosis). If you are, go to the ER.

Please drink plenty of water to keep yourself well hydrated.

If you are on insulin, you can increase your pre-meal insulin by 20-30%, and up to 100% if needed, and continue the sliding scale for corrections. You must closely monitor your blood sugar.

If you are not able to get your sugar down, and if you have chest pain or shortness of breath, see your doctor immediately. This may indicate a more serious condition, such as a heart attack.

I started on a new batch of insulin, and now I cannot get my sugar down. What should I do?

You might need to call the pharmacy to see if they can give you another batch of insulin to try. Insulin from the manufacturer to you has traveled a long distance. Believe it or not, things happen during the journey. It is not uncommon to have "bad" insulin.

Sometimes, you may have an expired insulin, or it was not stored properly. Therefore, you always have to pay attention to the condition of each insulin and store your opened and unopened insulin as recommended. Discard unused or unfinished insulin pen and vial if expired or you see clumps in your insulin or discoloration. For any insulin containing NPH (N), you need to mix well before you give the shot, but do not shake it.

I am going to have colonoscopy or day-surgery. Should I take my insulin and how should I take it?

Please read my other book <<Diabetes Questions and Answers More Than 400 Diabetes Frequently Asked Questions>>. I have a chapter discussing many aspects about dealing this situation. Colonoscopy is recommend to everybody over age of 50. All diabetes have to deal with it sooner or later. It is available on Amazon.com and other major bookstores.

.

Chapter 17. Final words-All about Insulin

Why should I not be afraid of insulin?

If used properly, insulin can help you. For type 1 diabetes, insulin allows you to live. For type 2 diabetes if used properly, it can reduce glucotoxicity and allow your beta cells to recover. Insulin can also be dangerous. It has lots of side effects like fluid retention, heart failure, hypokalemia, and might be linked to increased risk of cancer.

How can we reduce insulin use?

I have the following recommendations for you:

➢ Try your best to eat right. You need to take this seriously. Eating is the key for diabetes control. If your eating is not controlled, diabetes cannot be controlled, and then your insulin dose will need to be increased. Many studies have shown that a whole-food, plant-based diet can completely reverse diabetes and free you from your insulin demands if you have a type 2 diabetes.
➢ Keep yourself active. This is only 20%; 80% is diet. If possible, having a walk before and after a meal will help lower your insulin needs. This will also help "blood flow" and you will think better and feel more energized.

➤ Keep yourself well-hydrated. Dehydration increases insulin resistance and increases insulin needs.
➤ Know when to reduce your dose, like when you are expecting to do more strenuous exercise or physical work.
➤ Coping with your stress. Stress increases your insulin resistance and your insulin needs. You can try counseling, medications, and most importantly, activities like Taqi, Yoga.
➤ Use in combination with other medications like GLP-1 agonist or SGLT2 inhibitors.
➤ Do not just rely on insulin even if you have type 1 diabetes.

Anything else can I do to make my insulin use safer?

➤ Always check your sugars and have a plan so you are always prepared.
➤ Try to have a scheduled life as much as possible. If you have a chaotic lifestyle, you can expect to have troubles with insulin.
➤ If possible, always live with somebody. In case of an emergency, there is someone to help you give an emergency glucagon shot and call 911.
➤ Learn as much as you can about the insulin you are taking. The more you know, the better off you will be.
➤ If possible, try to get a CGM (continuous glucose monitor).
➤ If you are qualified, try to get a close-loop insulin pump.
➤ If you live on top of your diabetes, you can have a very positive and productive life. Many people are living a productive life while on insulin.

www.ingramcontent.com/pod-product-compliance
Lightning Source LLC
Chambersburg PA
CBHW052313220526
45472CB00001B/105

9 781979 935647